614 WAT £17.99

Public Health in Practice

ca   entre Libr

D0320100

Public Health in Practice

Edited by

Andrew Watterson

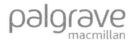

First published 2003 by
PALGRAVE MACMILLAN
Houndmills, Basingstoke, Hampshire RG21 6XS and
175 Fifth Avenue, New York, N.Y. 10010
Companies and representatives throughout the world

PALGRAVE MACMILLAN is the global academic imprint of the Palgrave
Macmillan division of St. Martin's Press, LLC and of Palgrave Macmillan Ltd.
Macmillan® is a registered trademark in the United States,
United Kingdom and other countries. Palgrave is a registered trademark
in the European Union and other countries.

ISBN 0–333–94617–0 paperback

This book is printed on paper suitable for recycling and made from fully
managed and sustained forest sources.

A catalogue record for this book is available from the British Library.

10   9   8   7   6   5   4   3   2   1
12   11   10   09   08   07   06   05   04   03

Printed and bound in Great Britain by
Creative Print & Design (Wales), Ebbw Vale

Contents

List of Figures, Boxes and Tables

Figure

Boxes

Tables

List of Contributors

Isobel Anderson works in the Housing Policy and Practice Unit, Stirling University in Scotland. She is also a member of the Chartered Institute of Housing and has worked in housing practice in the United Kingdom.

Aileen Barclay also works in the Housing Policy and Practice Unit, Stirling University, and has a background in learning disabilities and mental health.

Paul Belcher works in Environmental Sciences at the University of Wales Institute, Cardiff (UWIC), specialising in Housing and Public Health Policy. He has been an Environmental Health Officer (EHO) in South Wales.

Steve Bell is Health Promotion Manager at the Highland Health Board in Inverness, Scotland.

Yvonne Dalziel is a public health practitioner in the Lothian region of Scotland and she is also a 'community nurse'.

Maureen Dennis is a community health campaigner in Boston, Lincolnshire.

Thomas Gorman is a welfare rights advisor and community campaigner in Glasgow and the Clyde and visiting researcher at Stirling University.

Peter McCalister is a general practitioner at Bonnybridge in Scotland and Associate Advisor in continuing professional development for GPs in Forth Valley.

James McCourt works at Inverclyde Advice and Employment Centre and with PHASE TWO, a community action group on the Clyde.

John Middleton is Director of Public Health at Sandwell in the West Midlands, England and a public health physician.

Gary Mumford is a district EHO working in the City of Southampton. He also holds a degree in Psychology.

Colin Powell is in Environmental Sciences at UWIC and worked at the Welsh Health Promotion Authority and in health authorities.

Julie Prowse works in Health Studies at Bradford University. She specialises in health service and human resource management and international health issues.

Andrew Watterson works on health effectiveness and public health at Stirling University and is a registered occupational health and safety practitioner.

Jenny Watterson is a paediatric physiotherapist/primary care clinical specialist and visiting researcher at Stirling University looking at lay/professional knowledge.

John Wildsmith works in Environmental Sciences at UWIC and heads its Centre for Health, Safety and Environment. He has been an EHO in England.

Acknowledgements

Many thanks go to all the contributors to the book. Thanks too to Kate Niven and Tommy Starrs at Stirling University for providing such a friendly and stimulating work setting. Special thanks to the community groups in Chesterfield, Lincolnshire, Clydeside and the Highlands and Islands who provided a critical insight into why further public health advances are needed and why they should be at the heart of the process. Finally, especial thanks to Jon Reed and the Palgrave staff for their tolerance and help.

List of Abbreviations

AHPs	Allied health professionals such as physiotherapists, occupational therapists, speech therapists and radiographers. The term replaces PAMs
DEFRA	Department of Environment, Food and Rural Affairs
DFID	Department for International Development
DoH	Department of Health
DoT	Department of Transport
DsPH	Directors of Public Health
EEA	European Environment Agency
EH	Environmental health
EHIA	Environmental health impact assessment
EHO	Environmental Health Officer
EIA	Environmental imapct assessment
FAO	Food and Agriculture Organisation
FHSAs	Family Health Service Authorities
GPs	General Practitioners
HA	Health Authority
HAZ	Health Action Zones
HIA	Health Impact Assessment
HoN	Health of the Nation Report
HSE	Health and Safety Executive
HFA	WHO Health For All programmes
LHCC	Local Health Care Co-operative – only in Scotland
MOH	Medical Officer of Health
NHS	National Health Service
OHAC	UK tripartite occupational health advisory committee
OHN	Our Healthier Nation report
PCG	Primary Care Group
PCT	Primary Care Trust
PH	Public health
RHA	Regional Health Authority

RIPHH   Royal institution of Public Health and Hygiene
RSI   Repetitive strain injury
SAPs   Structural Adjustment Programmes
TLVs   Threshold Limit Values for chemicals
VWF   Vibration-induced whitefinger
WHO   World Health Organisation

1

Introduction

Andrew Watterson

The aims of the text

This book aims to locate and shed light on public health practice in a number of ways, primarily with regard to the role and function of public health professionals. The book also explores the interactions of public health professionals with other professionals, with users and communities and with public health bodies in the United Kingdom, and beyond. Effective public health practice should ensure that there are no neglected or hidden populations and all groups should be reached, albeit at times with different resources and staffing commitment.

The book investigates the public health practice of some specific professional groups through the eyes of those professionals. These professionals raise a range of technical, scientific, medical, policy and organisational issues about their work. It is a time of rapid change in UK health services and the challenges and opportunities for public health are many. For instance, there are important decisions to be taken about health priorities, health effectiveness, clinical effectiveness, the value of screening and how to involve the public in health planning. These subjects often present major political, economic, ethical and sometimes legal challenges

(Bradley and Burls 2000). The book does not seek to evaluate public health practice: others have attempted to do that (Muir Gray 1997; Atkin *et al.* 1999; Griffiths and Hunter 1999). It is not a manual on what to do. The book seeks to identify and analyse current concerns, debates and practice in public health from the key practitioner's perspective. The book also provides an opportunity to explore various facets of public health and view the inter-relationship or at times the separation of the various public health functions through the eyes of the different practitioners.

Public health can be as much about 'process' as content. The process draws on methods used to assess health threats and injuries as well as risks, to engage the public, to communicate information, to consult lay and professional groups in policy making and then to inform application of relevant technical skills. Such methods overlap, often a great deal. Some of the methods used by public health professionals, especially those that have frequently been undervalued or neglected in the past are discussed in Chapter 2. Health promoters and environmental health staff are for instance concerned with the process of community development. Everyone in public health at one level or another is concerned with the public, patients and their families. The National Health Service (NHS) has recently established a 'Consumers in NHS Research Support Unit' to examine these concerns more closely and to explore and represent user views in recognition that users are at the heart of public health concerns. This is the core of much innovative public health work. Some methods needed to ensure better public participation in public health go back over a hundred years, have been tested from 1920s and now involve citizens juries, town meetings along with other types of participatory involvement and focus groups (Stewart *et al.* 1994). The reality of community participation in the NHS is, however, still problematic whereas the rhetoric has been strong (Dockery 1996).

What is public health?

A plethora of terms and definitions have been used to describe the work of a range of public health 'practitioners'. These have included sanitary science, community hygiene, community health, community medicine, the 'old public' health', preventive medicine, social medicine and 'new public health'. A publication on public health practice should make explicit to the reader what sort of 'public health' is being practised. The various contributors to this book offer a range of views and explanations of public health that inform their particular practice. The 'new public health' emerged during the 1914–18 War and has been refined and revised ever since. By 1988, some of its most imaginative and energetic proponents viewed it as 'an approach which brings together environmental change and personal preventive measures with appropriate therapeutic interventions especially for the elderly and disabled. However, the New Public Health goes beyond an understanding of human biology and recognises the importance of those social aspects of health problems which are caused by lifestyles. In this way it seeks to avoid the trap of blaming the victim' (Ashton and Seymour 1988: 21). This approach has much to commend it as lifestyles are socially, economically and politically constructed and it informs many of the later contributions in this book.

The definition that follows, however, has guided the editor most strongly in the preparation of this book. It takes account of both old and new threats to public health and looks at the conditions of people in the context of their wider populations. It also clearly flags up the role of society in public health practice.

> Public health is what we, as a society, do to assure the conditions for people to be healthy. This requires that continuing and emerging threats to the health of the public be successfully countered. These include immediate crises, such as the AIDS epidemic, enduring problems such as the ageing of our population and the toxic products of a modern economy, transmitted through air, water, soil or food. (Committee for the Study of the Future of Public Health Washington, USA 1988)

History of public health

Public health, it could be argued, has always existed where there have been organised communities and was being practised long before industrialisation in the northern and western regions of the world (Table 1.1). Greek and Roman public health work has for instance been well documented. The breadth and pace of developments in public health did, however, widen and quicken in the nineteenth century Britain and North America

Table 1.1   A history of public health in the United Kingdom: from the Victorian times to the present day

Event and year	Key features
Chadwick report 1842 after cholera epidemics Sir John Simon, First chief medical officer, 1854. Snow on cholera, Farr, Victorian public health acts (Farrow S, 1988; Rosen, 1993)	Health problems due to poor housing and unsanitary conditions Appoint independent district medical officer. '*The interests of health and the interests of common physical convenience are in various cases identical*'. Recommends measures to improve housing, provide clean water and sanitation. PH responsibility of local authorities, MOsH appointments – but many not appointed until early 1900s
'Lloyd George' National Insurance Act 1909	Health insurance cover – for working men only. Women and children's health dealt with by local authority gift and charities
1948 NHS	Universal health care provision. Tripartite health system: hospital regional boards, GPs, local authorities responsible for PH; community nursing, environmental health, social services, generally under MOH
1974 NHS reorganisation	Unified health service. Social care/ environmental health remains with local authorities. PH doctors become community physicians. System of 'consensus management': any senior manager could veto Decisions
1976 Prevention and health – everybody's business' (DHSS, 1976)	Significant DoH and social security report – but prevention remained 'nobody's business'
1980 Black report on inequalities in health (DHSS, 1980)	Suppressed report on inequalities in health and health care destined to become very influential for the new PH. Proposed national interventions including child poverty eradication.
1982 NHS reorganisation based on Merrison report	Loss of area health authorities, still consensus management. FPCs responsible for GPs, other primary care contractors from 1984
1983 Griffiths report	General management introduced chief executive decision making
1980s New Public Health gains pace	PHA, unemployment and health groups. HFA, Transport/Health

Table 1.1 Continued

Event and year	Key features
1985 Targets for health for all in Europe agreed and published. (WHOEURO, 1985)	WHOEURO effort to make Global Health for all strategy relevant to Europe. Influential in UK local authorities seeking to implement such strategies. European healthy cities project started, Liverpool, Belfast, Glasgow, London UK collaborating centres.
1987 Health divide report (Whitehead, 1987)	Confirms widening health gap between rich and poor in 6 years following Black
1988 Acheson Report on Public Health in England (DoH, 1988)	Response predominantly to infectious disease scandals in hospitals, salmonella in eggs. Proposed Regional and District DsPH with clearer executive responsibility, Consultants in Communicable Diseases. Epidemiological resource expanded at all levels. Annual PH report re-introduced as strategic health planning vehicle. Restated DPH responsibility for local authority and local partner advice on healthy public policy
1990 Working for patients NHS White paper (DoH, 1990)	Purchaser/provider split with the 'internal market for health care' 'money follows patients' 'success rewarded'. NHS hospital trusts in keeping with the times completely ignored community services and later had to acknowledge need for community, and ambulance, NHS trusts. Family Health Services Authorities given greater powers in managing new GP contract
1991 The Health of the Nation (DoH, 1991)	Ist English health promotion targets and national attempt to set targets for health improvement. Fails to acknowledge economics influences on health and role of social, educational, economic policies to promote health; over emphasises health service as agent for delivery.
1996 Reorganisation	Redrew regional boundaries; merged NHS trust performance management and formed Regional Offices of the NHS, under civil service. Health authorities merged with FHSAs.
1998 English Health Action Zones set up (HAZs)	11 HAZs set up in small towns and large conurbations addressing urban and rural health inequalities. 26 zones set up covering

Table 1.1   Continued

Event and year	Key features
	40% of England's deprived populations. Aim to modernise health service and patient experience. Innovative programme in employment, housing and health related activity. Ist national policy worldwide to target deprivation and health. Unlike healthy cities has resources, is performance managed. Minister's interest on wane 3 years into the programme.
1998 A First class service (DoH, 1998) 1999 Health Act	Health improvement/ health inequality reduction become express NHS aims for first time. NHS has to do some good not just balance the books and stay out of trouble! PCGs set up in HAs. GPs to be part of HAs, work in primary care development, commissioning secondary care services, tackling health inequalities. Fundamental platform for PH intervention lost in favour of responsible GP list population. Clinical governance developed to improve standards: a managerial/systems issue not just about clinical performance 'creating an environment in which clinical excellence can flourish'
1998 Our healthier nation (OHN) green paper 1999 White paper (DoH, 1999)	Restates national health policy aims – to 'improve health and reduce inequalities in health' in 3 settings: neighbourhoods, workplaces and schools. 4 main problems – CHD and strokes, cancers, mental health, accidents. Announced resources for PH modernisation setting up Health Development Agency, PH observatories, training for multidisciplinary public health, especially in nursing, more funding for research
2000 Local government modernisation Act. Neighbourhood renewal and management	New duty of wellbeing – chance for new partnership wellbeing companies to pursue range of PH ventures? Local strategic partnerships and neighbourhood management to develop
2000 NHS plan (DoH, 2000)	Health improvement, health inequalities relegated to Ch 13. Partnership agenda for health improvement in OHN restated.

Table 1.1 Continued

Event and year	Key features
	Voluntary/community sector/ health needs of children omitted. Patient experience priority will be detrimental to health improvement in the long term
2001 lst UK national targets for reducing health inequalities. Same subject debated in Europe	Political priority for reducing inequalities confirmed and welcome recognition of cross-cutting nature of policy responses required at national, regional and local level.
2001 Shifting the balance of power DoH document	4 regional directors of health and social care created, regional DsPH in 9 government offices, 28 strategic health authorities and approximately 300 PCTs. PCT brief remains to improve health, improve primary health care
National strategy for infectious disease; creation of the National infection control and health protection agency (NICHPA) (DoH, 2002)	and commission hospital and specialised services. PCTs to lead PH positively – therefore 300 specialists/directors of PH rather than 90. Negative: will there only be 300 specialists? Inevitable fracturing of specialised PH services. Most PCTs too small to support all required skills. Organised for health services management benefit not discrete populations served by local strategic partnerships. Opportunity to develop non-specialist PH disciplines – community nursing – and potentially turn primary care into a PH morbidity information engine. Fracturing of infection control from mainstream local PH and local authorities. Health protection infection control, radiation, chemical incidents management agency created – now sleep safer in our beds? Immunisation programmes, food safety, local outbreak control, local infection control knowledge and management threatened.

Source: Middleton 2002.

(Fee and Acheson 1991: 1). It is important to understand where we have come from if we wish to plan effective public health for the future and practitioners such as John Ashton have used historical material to benchmark their own and other's progress in the field. John Middleton's table above provides one comprehensive view of key public health changes from the perspective of a public health physician and brings developments into the twenty-first century.

Threats to public health

Globally there are both old and new threats to public health through infectious diseases, war, the impact of global warming, economic instability and recession, food insecurity and water scarcity (McMichael 2001). The world's population has grown from one billion in 1900 to six billion in 2000. The world population is ageing and so presents critical public health challenges. If life expectancy is used as the sole criterion for public health successes, there has been a global success with average expectancy, according to World Health Organisation (WHO), increasing from 48 years in 1955 to a predicted 73 years in 2025. Child mortality figures have also improved with 21 million children dying before their fifth birthday in 1955 whereas in 1995, the figure was 11 million (Garrett 2001: 390). Sometimes a strange determinism manifests itself in national public health circles and these figures are presented as evidence that public health is improving *and* will continue to do so. These are also successes that conceal enormous human tragedy. National public health data reveal differences and major failures: in late 1990s, Malawi's average life expectancy rate was lower than in the 1930s and in Russia 'some regional downturns (in public health) were proportionally greater than anything witnessed during peacetime since the pneumonic plague reached Moscow in the fourteenth century' (Garrett 2001: 390).

In Central and Eastern Europe there has been a rapid worsening of the overall health of the public in particular countries and in Africa and parts of Asia the expected public health progress has not been realised. Major challenges to public health like malaria, HIV, TB and childhood mortality from waterborne diseases – technically easily solved – remain unmet. All too often, globally and nationally, some populations remain hidden in terms of public health needs. The global public health needs of the mentally ill or those with learning disabilities are addressed by relatively few public health practitioners and often remain neglected and marginalised as do the public health needs of the disabled, migrant workers and migratory populations. Globally, the health of women remains sorely neglected although some agencies such as WHO and within the United Kingdom Department for International Development (DFID) do position women and children at the centre of their development and health programmes. This book cannot cover every important and disparate threat to public health. Mental health is for instance touched on in the chapters dealing with housing and occupational health. Sexual health and substance abuse is touched on in the health promotion chapter. Food quality issues are discussed later in this chapter and in the chapters dealing with public health medicine, environmental health, health promotion and the conclusion. Poverty, including its impacts on health, is alluded to throughout the book. The chapters on primary care, public health medicine and occupational health raise questions about resources allocation, health economics and cost and risk benefit analysis.

In addition, it has been suggested that the significance and influence of public health should be extended to sectors of our society often viewed as discrete economic activities with no role to play on public health. For instance, persuasive arguments have been advanced for health to be the key to new farming and food policies in the United Kingdom. Here for instance dealing with food poisoning has been prioritised at a cost of just £1 billion a year whereas 'the costs of coronary vascular disease alone are around £10 billion a year (and) rising obesity in England suggests that the cost of such diet-related diseases will rise' (Lang and Rayner 2002). Lang argues that public health perspectives need to be emphasised far more when looking at the impact of the globalisation of food production and distribution (Lang 1998). In the past the contribution of Irish labourers to UK public health in the nineteenth century through construction work on sewers, water supplies and housing was seriously underestimated and grossly under-recorded. To avoid similar omissions perhaps we should recognise the contributions to healthy food production, both positive and negative, of agricultural workers and farmers to the public's health. Equally the public health impacts on employees of working conditions in the agricultural and food industries should not be neglected (Watterson 2000).

Challenges for public health

The globalisation of public health presents enormous opportunities, threats and challenges for public health advances. For example, some questionable global 'public health entrepreneurs' are touting for trade, just as arms traders do, outside their own countries when the wares (both methods and policies) they are selling have not been evaluated or barely evaluated within their own countries. In this context the role of what might be pejoratively called the 'public health industry' is worthy of examination. All professional groups may operate restrictive practices and can be highly defensive. All professional groups may protect their own interests for reasons relating to status, security, career and salary structure. Yet, public health is as much about democracy, empowerment, accountability, transparency and communication as it is about professional scientific skills. Recent public health plans and charters from the United Kingdom and WHO have prioritised transparent practice and highlighted the central position of user, consumer and community involvement in public health planning. Public health workers are often advocating action that, if effective, could dispense with their services: an unlikely outcome but a potentially threatening one for those workers. Outside Europe and North America, there are also pressures to use community workers rather than physicians or nurses to achieve public health progress: again real threats to two of the biggest health professional groups.

These new developments and challenges encompass and envisage a wider span of public health influences in order to make particular interventions effective. This bigger picture has been explored and advocated in the United Kingdom over many years but the message has rarely reached politicians at central or local government level and, where it did, was rarely taken on board. Hence the neglect by politicians of the work of Mayhew documenting poverty and related adverse health effects in the nineteenth century, Booth doing the same thing at the beginning of the twentieth century and Rowntree and others following down similar routes. By 1930s, medical officers of health and sanitary inspectors – now called environmental health officers- were collaborating to describe the consequences of poverty, poor nutrition and unemployment on health (M'Gonigle and Kirby 1936).

Reports on Inequalities in Health in the 1980s began to expand the earlier poverty work and provide indisputable evidence of the adverse effects of poverty. Others working in public health in the late 1980s and early 1990s provided more detailed accounts of these effects linked to the new public health, including gender as well as class; commercial as well as industrial drivers affecting public health. In addition personal lifestyle factors were linked to community health initiatives and healthy cities work (Martin and McQueen 1989). The new public health agenda has been most graphically described by a public health physician and a health promoter in Liverpool (Ashton and Seymour 1988). They moved away from the simplistic lifestyle and victim-blaming of some of the UK government's policies of the 1980s and sought to incorporate old public health concerns – housing, water supply, unadulterated food – with policies that tackled new public health problems such as AIDS and substance use and to link these with WHO Health For All and Healthy Cities objectives and community development techniques. By 1991, major efforts were underway to focus on significant public health interventions, including tackling the tobacco industry, the arms trader, international economics and third world debt: all in the context of the role of public policy (Draper 1991). These policy concerns have been re-iterated by more recent international commentators on the global public health position (Beaglehole and Bonita 1997).

The solutions to public health problems?

The first dedicated public health minister in the United Kingdom was only appointed in the late 1990s, some considerable time after ministers for fisheries and roads. This followed a period of national public health planning that resulted in many targets and objectives being set through the 'Health of the Nation' strategy (Sec. State 1992). These strategies, however, could either not be delivered or were effectively derailed by pressures from the powerful acute health sector. Treating disease rather than promoting public health is still the 'de facto' policy priority of much of the NHS in response to public concerns and perceived electoral pressures. Where public health has been flagged up during the last decades of the twentieth century, lifestyle approaches to public health have sometimes displaced life circumstance approaches. There has, however, recently been another welcome shift in England through the 'Our Healthier Nation' strategy with wide governmental recognition of the central role of socio-economic factors influencing health (DoH 1998). How the tensions and shifts on poverty and health – loosening corporation tax on companies and having an underfunded health service for instance – will work through in practice and whether resources will be effectively redirected to the poor in the United Kingdom and improve public health has yet to be established (Shaw *et al.* 1999).

In some fields public health responses have been skewed and proved problematic and resistant to community concerns with a mismatch between professional and public perceptions of risk and harm. For instance, suggestions that occupational hazards such as asbestos or environmental pollution such as water pollution at Camelford could be major factors in the disease patterns of particular populations have often been dismissed. Lifestyle, smoking and dietary habits have been proposed not simply as primary but sometimes the sole causes of diseases. We continue to await condemnations of government policies by government ministers across the world for their failures to take rapid and effective action against tobacco companies, alcohol companies and the transport industry for their role in the production of enormous quantities of known major carcinogens and the exposure of large sections of the world's populations to such substances. We await tabloid campaigns for citizens to protest outside the homes of company directors and former health ministers for working in or supporting the arms, tobacco, drink and food industries that cause hundreds of thousands of deaths each year in Europe alone. Such campaigns would ensure that the major causes and the major culprits of preventable diseases were identified.

However, with the warp and weft of both governmental and professional policies, it is possible to find effective public health operating in a myriad of ways despite many tensions and contradictions. The move, on paper if not in practice, towards exploring wider dimensions of influence in establishing the root causes of disease has been widely welcomed. A UK Minister of Health recently stated that public health improvements 'were all to do with transport, housing and so on' (Clarke 2001). When wider public health issues have been neglected for decades by governments because of both vested economic interests and the domination of the disease focussed NHS by hospitals and acute care needs, such ministerial interventions are welcome.

The medicalisation of public health issues has in the past served to explain albeit partially the failure to advance upstream public health approaches and related to the workings of a narrow 'medical model' which is now almost entirely absent in the UK public health teams. The tensions between medical and non-medical models of public health, including research and training, are well understood and the limits of the former and the development difficulties of the latter have been explored, but with no real solutions proffered, in academic and research settings (Gabbay 1999: 266–7).

All the UK NHS and regional directors of public health are physicians and this has led to the debate about the value and indeed the evidence base for effective practice for such a phenomenon (McPherson 2001). Attempts to assess the best type of public health team, the constitution and location of that team within either the health, local authority, education sectors or across all sectors are complex. These issues are addressed more fully in the chapters within the book. In the United Kingdom 'professional' public health work has diversified in England, Wales, Scotland and Northern Ireland. There are now some organisational and support differences between the four countries. For instance in England, the primary care groups and trusts in the NHS have been given a public health role relating to reducing health inequalities; addressing social, economic and environmental influences on health and promoting health in places such as schools and workplaces (Gillam *et al.* 2001).

A serious worry amongst many public health physicians is that public health teams, currently working at a regional level and already frequently under-staffed, may now be fragmented and spread so thinly in the Primary Care Trusts (PCTs). PCTs may lack developed public health and epidemiology awareness, that they will not function effectively (Dobson 2001). This may reflect the overwhelming influence of political, social and economic factors in public health that can swamp the commitment and technical skills and commitment of dedicated public health professionals.

The Nongovernmental Organisations (NGOs) have played and continue to play a significant lobbying, campaigning, training and education role in public health. Professional bodies such as the Faculty of Public Health Medicine, the Chartered Institute of Environmental Health, the Institute of Housing and the Institution of Occupational Safety and Health may adopt an advocacy, lobbying and an educational role. NGOs such as the UK Public Health Alliance, committed and focussed on campaigning, as are broad-based. Bodies such as Oxfam, Save the Children, Greenpeace and Friends of the Earth may also have both general and specific public health objectives. They may employ public workers on public health projects within and outside the United Kingdom linked to housing, food, water and health programmes or to communication, campaigning and education work.

US public health researchers have stressed the adverse effects of war on public health but this issue has been relatively neglected by the world's most prosperous countries as also have the global mortality figures relating to polluted water or infectious agents. If a nation's economy benefits from arms sales that threaten public health or a country's pharmaceutical industries benefit from selling expensive drugs to developing countries or a nation can dump its old products and toxic waste cheaply in developing countries, it seems that public health all too often takes second place to national or multi-national economic self-interest. Following the September 11th 2001 attack on the World Trade Centre in New York, some aspects of the public health effects of war have risen in the agenda. Increased US research and funding has now been devoted to 'bioterrorism'. Yet this is in a country which in 2000 had more than 44 million citizens who lacked any health insurance at all – mostly African-American, Hispanic and poor white people and whose public health system faced major challenges (Garrett 2001: 8). The public health war on disease and death is moving in and out of the shadows of the War on Terrorism debate but all too often remains in darkness especially when the politics of disease-treatment means that northern hemisphere secondary and tertiary care continues to consume the vast amount of global health resources.

Themes and subjects

The themes that flow through the book relate to multi-disciplinary and inter-disciplinary approaches to public health in the United Kingdom and beyond. The prime movers in public health were perceived as 'health professionals' for much of the nineteenth and twentieth centuries. These were physicians and nurses working in hospital, lab and community settings and sanitary inspectors now called environmental health officers. What these public health professionals attempt to do is at the centre of the book. The roles of public health workers as technicians, facilitators, advocates or evangelists are covered as are some of the equity and ethical public health practice challenges. The conclusion is produced by a group that contains users of public health who have their own perspective on the effectiveness, responsiveness, relevance, transparency and accountability of the discipline.

The book therefore focusses on the practice of a number of the key professional groups who for the most part impact upon public health directly. Public health physicians still lead public health practice in health authorities often supported by health promotion staff, non-medical public health specialists, statisticians, infection control nurses and technical support staff. In local authorities, environmental health officers will play the key public health role in food safety, housing, pollution control – air, water and noise – within local authority jurisdiction and again may operate in departments containing technical staff, occupational health and health promotion practitioners.

Public health nursing has a long history in the United Kingdom with health visitors, fever nurses, nurses working in acute settings whose patients were affected by public health problems in the nineteenth century, district nurses, school nurses and practice nurses. Such nursing specialisms have relied on often unique direct contact with patients and communities that have given them a central public health role not always acknowledged by others. The public health nurse is now developing more extensive strategic and support roles in some regions within the United Kingdom. Nurses and midwives have also become part of the 'barefoot doctor' workforce in some countries. 'Barefoot doctors' are often key public health and primary health care workers where permanent access to health care is lacking which means much of the world (Stark 1985). They may or may not have a non-health professional background but they have been playing a major international role in public health in Africa, Asia and the Middle East over several decades.

General practitioners (GPs), sometimes called family doctors outside the United Kingdom, have always had an important but frequently understated and under-explored role to play in public health and are the first medical point of contact and for many the only medical point of contact for the public for most of their lives. The movement of public health professionals into primary care trusts may provide the ultimate and certainly a major challenge to the practice of public health in the United Kingdom. At the heart of this activity are GPs, practice nurses, health visitors, district nurses and midwives linked to other allied health professional groups. The inter-relationship between acute hospital services, primary care and the value of connecting acute care with public health is, however, relatively under-explored. Nurses, allied health professionals (AHPs who used to be called professions allied to medicine) such as dieticians, physiotherapists, occupational therapists, speech therapists and podiatrists and medical staff are beginning to look more closely at these inter-relationships in the context of mother, baby and child support, improving care of coronary heart care patients in the community and the general move to reduce bed blocking and pressures on hospital acute services through better and more effective public health and community care interventions. GP interventions in conjunction with practice nurses, allied health professional groups such as midwives and health visitors and district nurses and, in Scotland, and elsewhere in the world with WHO family health nurse can make potentially major contributions to public health.

Housing policy and practice reflects good public health in terms of creating a healthy environment through planning, development and building of homes and preventing ill-health through proper maintenance of homes, support for householders and related infrastructure for communities nationally and internationally. This links in with environmental health and economic policy matters. Occupational health addresses an area of human activity that affects at least one-third of most people's adult lives and may involve work-related effects too, as well as occupationally caused diseases, with direct and often long-term impacts on environmental health, psycho-social health and musculo-skeletal health. Occupational health and safety can include major public health issues not only from the physical and organisational impacts of work but also from threats such as transport to and from work, pollution and diet, exercise and lifestyle choices whilst at work.

Promoting good health through effective interventions with individuals, groups, communities and the public has always been viewed as a very desirable activity but how to educate, inform and intervene in such matters has proved perhaps one of the largest challenges for those working in public health. Many public health professionals who are not specialist health promoters will draw on this discipline in their practice as the later chapters by the public health nurse, the public health physician and environmental health officers reveal.

Finally, economic and policy matters may well determine the success of small-scale, regional, national and international public health interventions. This is why the influences on international health are covered in a separate chapter in the book and the issue discussed there in many respects do underpin everything else in the book.

Each author has presented her or his independent view of public health practice. They speak for themselves and their views are not necessarily shared by other authors in the book. There may be different tensions, different challenges and opportunities presented in each chapter but there are also common themes and often common approaches and shared methodologies. Responses may be more or less shaped by government policy – political, economic and social; by international and regional developments; by different sets of perceptions and different guidelines.

Many of the debates relate as much to social, economic and political values as they do to 'evidence'. Evidence-based health care is central to public health (Muir Gray 1997). However, at times such evidence may be presented as unproblematic and accepted uncritically. For instance, Cochrane Systematic reviews may be accepted as entirely authoritative and scientific when there may be all sorts of value judgements and pressures – direct and indirectly – influencing their authors. In 2002, leading US public health researchers have directly raised the problem of both government agencies and academic centre staff providing the scientific base for policy decisions whilst 'they are also subject to efforts to politicise or silence objective scientific research. Such actions increasingly use sophisticated and complex strategies that put evidence-based policy making at risk' (Rosenstock and Jackson Lee 2002: 14).

Rosenstock and Jackson Lee revealed a picture that is replicated in many parts of the globe and should prompt a very careful scrutiny by public health practitioners of the evidence base that they use. For instance, they cite work showing that 60 per cent of non-industry studies on selected chemicals – alachlor, atrazine, formaldehyde and perchloroethylene – found the chemicals hazardous whilst only 14 per cent of industry-sponsored studies did. Of 70 review articles on the use of calcium-channel antagonists, 96 per cent of authors supportive of their use had financial links with companies making these products whereas the figure for non-company authors was 60 per cent and for critical authors it was 37 per cent. Similar figures for review articles on the health effects of passive smoking found 74 per cent of authors critical of such a link had tobacco industry affiliations. The politics of knowledge production provides a rather different context to some aspects of public health research evidence that may be used to underpin practice or guide national and international public health policies.

Common themes in the book include:

- The benefits of public health – social, economic, physical and psycho-social.
- Partnerships between communities and public health professionals – what they are and how they have been or should be achieved.
- Partnerships between health professional groups: what works, what does not and why.
- How local players link with national, governmental and international players on the public health scene.
- How some of the root causes of ill health are addressed by public health professionals in such fields as social inequalities, poor housing, occupational health, primary care and environmental health.

Andrew Watterson and Jenny Watterson in Chapter 2 provide a summary and discussion of some of the major research tools available to those working in public health, how these tools have developed and what their strengths and weaknesses are. The benefits of bringing together a range of methods and sometimes new or neglected methodological thinking are explored linked to some of the types of public health work described in the following chapters.

Julie Prowse in Chapter 3 deals with the underpinning influence of international economic agencies and their policies on public health and provides evidence for the impact of macroeconomic policies on national and indeed regional and local public health strategies. At the centre is the enormous but not exclusive influence that poverty plays in damaging public health in 'developing' and 'developed countries'. Attempts to ameliorate the impacts of such policies and practices at a national or local level may prove very challenging but can make real public health impacts for communities.

John Middleton in Chapter 4 looks at the work of a Director of Public Health from the perspective of public health medicine and provides a rich insight into the activities of such a post. Measuring health problems, exploring interventions and seeking to ensure such interventions are at the core of the work. The medical, organisational and advocacy roles of the post are demonstrated in accounts of interventions on road traffic accidents, food policy development and health service and local government interfaces.

Yvonne Dalziel in Chapter 5 examines the expanding role of nursing in public health, the work of 'public health nursing' in a primary care and community context and highlights the relevance of community development approaches to that role. Strategic planning, alliance building and community empowerment are the critical approaches used to address health inequalities. This requires refocussing nursing groups such as health visitors even further towards a public health role. Facilitatory organisational structures are critical to the success of such a shift and the author concludes with reference to the new 'public health practitioner' posts – sometimes occupied by a nurse, sometimes not – now developed in some parts of the United Kingdom.

Peter McCalister in Chapter 6 looks at how public health issues and public health approaches are taken up by busy GPs, how current clinical problems relevant to public health are addressed and how the tensions and problems created at the primary care level are dealt with in conjunction with other medical and public health staff. This provides an insight into the primary care team and its links with disciplines such as health promotion. The chapter provides a wide range of examples of practice based on contrasting developments, training needs, public expectations and epidemiological evidence.

Isobel Anderson and Aileen Barclay in Chapter 7 carefully examine the direct and indirect influences of housing on public health and explore some of the strategies that may help to improve housing stock and suitability. This locates public health very much within a multi-sectoral approach and stresses the inter-relationship between governmental policy, central and local, and economic and political forces and the need for coherent thinking to make links between agencies. The problems faced by housing officials are addressed and some evidence of low cost, good public health solutions are provided partly influenced by such factors as climate and community development.

John Wildsmith, Colin Powell, Paul Belcher and Gary Munford in Chapter 8 cover the diverse work of environmental health and the expectations that exist for generalist environmental health officers in the United Kingdom. The breadth of their work in food hygiene, housing and pollution control is described and the critical policy options now open to them are illustrated. The community development aspects of their work again appear to be coming to the fore and their role as risk communicators, risk managers, risk assessors and facilitators is analysed. Their work overlaps with many other public health groups.

Andrew Watterson in Chapter 9 looks at occupational health and safety in the global and the UK contexts. He examines what the roles and function of occupational health and safety practitioners may be in order to tackle a major problem in public health. The practice entails technical, ethical and organisational activity; all of which are discussed. Partnership building is viewed as critical. Some of the tools and tensions involved in this work are analysed especially the use of the precautionary principle and best practices are suggested.

Steve Bell in Chapter 10 examines the role of health promotion in public health from the perspective of the health promotion specialist who works with health professional staff who have a general health promotion role. He provides an insight into the strategic and operational perspectives of a varied discipline and how it fits within a public health department and rolls out to primary care professionals, social workers, teachers and others. Illustrations are provided of health promotion practice in clinical settings and in community settings. The subject is 'downstream' but often provides the principal public health contact for individuals and communities on prevention of disease approaches.

Chapter 11 concludes the book with a synthesis and a call for public health to go further up the policy and politician's agenda but also for public health professionals to do even more not only to act as advocates and champions of public health but also to move forward at an even greater pace in developing public health with and by the public itself.

Guiding public health principles

Effective public health should be based on the WHO principles of 'upstream' health interventions to prevent the development of avoidable diseases rather than focus on 'downstream' medical interventions to treat preventable diseases. The achievement of such an approach should therefore rest on decision-making underpinned by the precautionary principle. For as Thomas Fuller observed 'He who cures a disease may be the skillfullest, but he that prevents it is the safest physician' (Legge 1934). The precautionary principle has been traced back to the Hippocratic Oath precept of doing no harm and this principle is now or should be a major driver in any effective public health approach. The precautionary principle requires that action should be taken to protect public health even when clear scientific evidence of harm is lacking. It further places the burden of proof of no harm on those proposing actions that may endanger public health (Geiser in Raffensperger and Tickner 1999: xxiii).

Such an approach provides the means to deal with scientific uncertainty and the impacts of technological and commercial development on public health. It reflects the wisdom of pursuing what has been termed a prudent pessimist approach – perhaps better named a prudent action approach – as against a scientific optimist's approach with all the risks and none of the benefits that entails. The former approach is 'expertist' and rooted in 'scientism' which tends to reflect a view of science and technology as all conquering and unproblematic with answers to all questions being possible if sufficient funding/resource is available. The latter approach is far more open, far more cautious and involves participation from those likely to be affected by developments as well as those researching the science. It looks to sustainable growth rather than no growth or growth at any cost. It builds in more careful concerns about public health, wider community and global concerns and the environment.

This book is about public health practice but where theoretical perspectives inform that practice or help us to understand that practice better, then they will be discussed. For as Tawney noted: 'The English are incurious as to theory, take fundamentals for granted, and are more interested in the state of the roads than in their place on the map' (Tawney 1961). Public health, new and old, needs to address the state of our roads and to locate itself on the map in terms of good practice underpinned by relevant evidence and methodologies. Effective practice should be grounded in a variety of critically appraised evidence bases, precautionary principle approaches and use meaningful theory to inform policy.

References

Ashton J and Seymour H (1988) *The New Public Health.* Open University Press, Milton Keynes.

Atkin K, Lunt N and Thompson C (1999) *Evaluating Community Nursing.* Bailliere Tindall, Edinburgh.

Beaglehole R and Bonita R (1997) *Public Health at the Crossroads: Achievements and Prospects.* Cambridge University Press, Cambridge.

Bradley P and Burls A (2000) *Ethics in Public and Community Health.* Routledge, London.

Clarke M (2001) End of term report for Alan Milburn. *BMJ* **323**: 290.

De Koning K and Martin M (1996) *Participatory Research in Health: Issues and Experiences.* Zed Books, London.

Department of Health (1998) *Our Healthier Nation.* HMSO, London.

Dobson R (2001) Primary care trusts to take lead on public health. *BMJ* **323**: 249.

Dockery G (1996) 'Rhetoric or reality? Participatory research in the NHS, UK' in De Koning and Martin (eds) *Participatory Research in Health: Issues and Experiences.* Zed Books, London, pp 164–76.

Draper P (ed.) (1991) *Health through Public Policy: The Greening of Public Health.* Greenprint, London.

Farrow S (ed.) (1988) *The Public Health Challenge.* Hutchinson with Faculty of Community Medicine of the Royal Colleges of Physicians UK.

Fee E and Acheson RM (1991) *A History of Education in Public Health.* Oxford University Press, Oxford.

Gabbay J (1999) 'The socially constructed dilemmas of academic public health' in Griffiths and Hunter (eds) *Perspectives in Public Health.* Radcliffe Medical Press, Abingdon, pp 261–8.

Garrett L (2001) *The Betrayal of Trust: The Collapse of Global Public Health.* Oxford University Press, Oxford.

Gillam S, Abbott S and Banks-Smith J (2001) Can primary care groups and trusts improve health? *BMJ* **323**: 89–92.

Griffiths S and Hunter D (1999) *Perspectives in Public Health.* Radcliffe Medical Press, Abingdon.

Lang T (1998) The new globalisation, food and health: is public health receiving its due emphasis? *J Epidemiol Community Health* **52**(9): 538–9.

Lang T and Rayner G (eds) (2002) *Why Health is the Key to the Future of Farming and Food.* Centre for Food Policy, Thames Valley University, London.

Legge T (1934) *Industrial Maladies.* Oxford University Press, Oxford.

Martin C and McQueen DV (eds) (1989) *Readings for a New Public Health.* Edinburgh University Press, Edinburgh.

McMichael A (2001) *Human Frontiers, Environments and Disease.* Cambridge University Press, Cambridge.

McPherson K (2001) Public Health does not need to be led by doctors. *BMJ* **322**: 1593–6.

M'Gonigle GCM and Kirby J (1936) *Poverty and Public Health*. Victor Gollancz Ltd, London.

Middleton J (2002) Chapter 4 in *Public Health in Practice*. Palgrave, Basingstoke.

Muir Gray JA (1997) *Evidence-based Health Care: How to Make Health Policy and Management Decisions*. Churchill Livingstone, Edinburgh.

Raffensperger C and Tickner J (1999) *Protecting Public Health and the Environment: Implementing the Precautionary Principle*. Island Press, Washington DC.

Rosen G (1993) *A History of Public Health*. Expanded edn. Johns Hopkins Press, Baltimore.

Rosenstock L and Jackson Lee L (2002) Attacks on science: the risks to evidence-based policy. *Am J Public Health* **92**(1): 14–18.

Secretary of State for Health (1992) *The Health of the Nation: A Strategy for Health in England*. HMSO, London.

Shaw M, Dorling D, Gordon G and Davey Smith G (1999) *The Widening Gap: Health Inequalities and Policy in Britain*. Policy Press, Bristol.

Stark R (1985) Lay workers in primary health care: victims in the process of social transformation. *Soc Sci Med* **20**(3): 269–75.

Stewart J, Kendall E and Coote A (1994) *Citizens Juries*. Institute for Public Policy Research, London.

Tawney RH (1961) *The Acquisitive Society*. Fontana, London.

Watterson A (2000) Agricultural science and food policy for consumers and workers: recipes for public health successes or disasters. *New Solutions* **10**(4): 317–24.

Whitehead M (1987) *The Health Divide*. Health Education Council, London.

2

Public Health Research Tools

Andrew Watterson and Jenny Watterson

Introduction

This chapter focuses on a small selection of the research methods available to public health practitioners, namely epidemiology, focus groups, participatory research including rapid appraisal, lay-worker and community epidemiology and health impact–health needs assessments. These research tools have been chosen for discussion because there is either much debate or much interest surrounding them, particularly how they might produce the types of evidence which can inform effective public health practice (Loader 1999; Davey Smith and Ebrahim 2001). This chapter does not aim to provide a crash course in research methods but rather to discuss the nature, usefulness and impact on communities of research methods and processes. Later chapters in the book will shed further light on research approaches and techniques briefly discussed here including methodological, technical, staffing and resources constraints. The emphasis will be on the practical application of knowledge and how lay groups can themselves explore public health in local and global contexts.

Public health researchers sometimes voice the view that unless their work is based on 'scientific' genetic, biochemical and pharmacological approaches, it is not considered rigorous or valued in scientific and medical communities. Other public health researchers may have been caught up in a search for professional credibility and status by concentrating on large and expensive quantitative epidemiological studies to the exclusion of other and sometimes complementary qualitative, participatory approaches that can inform effective everyday public health practice and outcomes. This situation may reflect the historically central role that physicians have played in UK public health and perhaps an erroneously self-perceived vulnerability regarding the value of non-positivist evidence when dealing with clinical and lab-based colleagues. These tensions are also somewhat sterile for much good public health practice is of course based on traditional research tools including lab-based research in pharmacology and to a lesser extent microbiology. The Public Health Laboratory Service still plays a pivotal role in public health surveillance and their work underpins many public health interventions down the line. However, it is not the intention of this book or of this chapter to explore these well established approaches and services but rather to discuss some alternative approaches through which effective public health practice can be informed. This book is about the production and application of different types of public health knowledge in practice rather than about public health in the laboratory.

Many UK public health teams are multi-disciplinary, potentially comprising of public health physicians, non-clinical public health specialists, nurses, health promotion staff, statisticians, non-clinical epidemiologists, dentists and pharmacists. In addition, staff such as police officers, who may focus on road traffic accidents or drug use problems, may be seconded and crucially, users should be part of the team. An excellent example of the value of lay-professional partnership-working in defining real-life issues and thereby producing the types of evidence that can both effectively inform solutions and obviate the theory practice gaps that inhibit so much practical and policy implementation, is that on child accidents research (Rice *et al.* in Popay and Williams 1994).

Each of these 'public health practitioner' groups may, both implicitly and explicitly, draw on specific theories, methodologies and methods and indeed pool methods to inform their practice. Public health research methods are therefore essentially eclectic. Beyond the medical, nursing and pharmacological methods traditionally employed by clinical public health staff, practitioners may also use technologically innovative tools such as acoustics for sound and vibration monitoring in workplaces and wider environmental settings alongside qualitative research tools which aim to gain experiential knowledge from the participants' (subjects') perspective. Health promoters and accident prevention researchers may use multi-media methods to gain useful knowledge, get public health messages across and to evaluate the impact of those messages so that approaches can be modified should they prove ineffective.

Public Health staff may develop and draw on methods acquired before or after their qualification and appointment in order to allow them to better address public health issues. These might include financial management and other methodological skills gained through MBA programmes or skills linked to policy analysis gained in MPH programmes. Educational, psychological and other social science approaches and statistical methods are influential in the work of both official and NGO public health organisations. However, it should also be remembered that the sort of approaches to public health that have succeeded best in the past are still, according to one of the United Kingdom's most active public health practitioners, relevant today. These core principles and values include 'an independent voice, appropriate research, production of reports, populism, advocacy, resourcefulness and pragmatism, the legitimacy of working locally, humanitarianism and a strong moral tone, cost-effectiveness of prevention, the need for organisation' (Ashton 1999: 26). Whilst technical approaches and support are now relatively widely available, what is missing are research methods courses and public health curricula that effectively train students in gaining and using an independent voice, using progressive rather than reactionary populism, and legitimate effective advocacy work and the adoption of a strong moral dimension for the collective benefit of the public health.

The critical questions are what are and who defines the issues and how can appropriate knowledge be gained and applied in practice. Effective Public Health teams choose the most suitable methodologies and methods primarily in the context of the issue to be addressed and the time, resources and skills, including those of the community, available to them. Effective Public Health should be based on the WHO principles of promoting 'upstream' health interventions to prevent the development of avoidable diseases rather than a traditional focus on 'downstream' medical interventions to treat preventable diseases. The achievement of such an approach should therefore rest on decision-making underpinned by the precautionary principle. The precautionary principle depends as much on informed social, economic and political reasoning as it does on science and medicine. Indeed for the nineteenth Century German medical practitioner, Rudolph Virchow, medicine was 'applied social science' (Rosen 1974: 62). Central to the approach is a need to assess the purpose and impact of any developments that might impinge on health in terms of environmental factors – be they personal, social or physical. In this context the first step in protecting public health should be the prevention of approval of dangerous substances or processes – be they in food, water, air, for domestic, leisure or workplace use. This should be achieved through rigorous toxicology or other scientific and technological testing. Later chapters in the book will shed further light on some of these issues.

Evidence-based public health?

'Evidence-based public health practice' aims to underpin and promote effective public health decision-making. The introduction above indicates that there is a range of types of evidence that can be produced and a diversity of views as to what counts as legitimate evidence (Jenkinson 1997; Bury and Mead 1998; Dawes *et al.* 1999). Evidence may constitute professionals' statistical or epidemiological reports from randomised control trials or nutritional studies or health services research (Muir Gray 1997). Evidence can also be qualitatively derived from the user/community perspective perhaps relating to the experienced effectiveness of a drug treatment or surgical intervention or equally to the effectiveness of information, education, counselling and support services to reduce unwanted early teenage pregnancies (Carter *et al.* 1999).

What counts as evidence may therefore include not only accurate epidemiological and clinical data but also qualitative and observational data from communities and health professionals about attitudes: what works and what does not work in public health interventions and why. It follows that there may be combinations of evidence that might support or reject public health approaches. For instance, biomedical evidence may fully support vaccinations but if other evidence demonstrates that public uptake of such vaccinations is declining or public confidence in that medical and scientific evidence is waning, then different public health strategies will be needed if practice is to be effective. Public health starts by understanding where the public is not where we might wish them to be.

It is also now widely but not universally accepted that: 'researchers should be aware that the choice of research question, the outcomes measured and the population on which the research is to be conducted all are value-laden decisions. It is not possible for researchers to be completely objective; therefore it is important for investigators to try to identify their own perspectives and values and to try and incorporate the perspectives and values of the population being researched' (Burls and Cabello-Lopez in Bradley and Burls 2000: 138).

It follows that debates about 'quantitative versus qualitative research methods' in public health are particularly futile and arid. However, the interface between professional/lay and theoretical/experiential knowledge in public health does indicate the need to understand some fundamental differences between quantitative and qualitative research methodologies: namely how the world is viewed and therefore how it might be studied. Traditionally, quantitative approaches are rooted in positivist philosophy which views the world as a single stable reality, as amenable to scientific enquiry as the natural sciences where only variables that can be objectively known through the senses and signified by language are considered scientifically testable to produce unfalsified knowledge (Popper 1959). Hence, quantitative methodologies emphasise technical methods by which these variables can be defined, isolated and then deductively tested. In contrast qualitative approaches are premised on an ontological assumption of a world of multiple experienced realities created through human interactions. Here, the way we think the world can be studied, epistemology, needs to take account of meaning, motive and action from individuals' situated perspectives (Cuff *et al.* 1990). Not only are context and the tacit dimensions of experience all important here but crucially for evidence-based public health practice, qualitative epistemologies create the possibilities for validating lay knowledge.

Hence, quantitative and qualitative methodologies are not directly comparable but rather these approaches and the research methods and tools they inform may be assessed as being more or less useful to the public health issues being addressed. Similarly, criteria of methodological rigour applied to all research to promote good, trustworthy evidence must be appropriate to the research methodology adopted. For qualitative approaches this includes locating research activity as a value-laden social event in itself and, as Burls and Cabello-Lopez (2000) note above, this requires investigators to make their own value positions explicit and to actively interrogate the influences this may have on the evidence produced. The concept of 'value-free' scientific research is not tenable.

Having set out our own value position the rest of this chapter will be devoted to brief commentary on some of the advantages and disadvantages of selected research tools and how these qualities can inform effective public health practice.

Biological, biochemical, microbiological, pharmacological research approaches

These traditional positivist approaches emphasise the importance of isolating the variables to be tested and measured with relationships between variables established as statistically significant creating generalisable knowledge. Quantitative methods and research findings in these fields have been critical to public health advances such as those dealing with infectious diseases. Interestingly some of these major achievements have been initiated by concerns to address basic socio-political problems relating to poverty, poor housing, water supply and food security.

Other research enquiries began after the affluent became concerned about the threats to their health from infectious diseases among the dispossessed: cholera in nineteenth Century United Kingdom demonstrates the self-interested motivation of the middle classes in supporting public health initiatives. Amelioration of these problems required policy actions in addition to the original scientific research. The successful application of quantitative health knowledge may therefore also need to draw on methods that explore complex interactions and promote partnerships between natural and social science methodologies. In mental health, for instance, there is a need to understand biological, pharmacological and also social science data. This locates and recognises the role of social context as well as biochemistry in influencing an individual's mental health problems and what might facilitate or inhibit effective intervention. Polarised debates about methods seem futile when in practice these differing types of evidence can be complementary.

Similarly, the idea of a moral and value free vacuum in research practice, where ethical considerations can merely be viewed as issues of process and 'informed consent', and the choice of research topic and use of the knowledge so produced is unrelated to anything, is defunct. Public health research and practice needs to locate traditional/quantitative evidence in the wider context of its use and acknowledge accountability for the implications of research activity. For example, ethical concerns with regard to the conduct and application of genetic research are morally significant. This is especially so when such research relates to susceptibility to a particular disease or environmental and occupational health insult and the identification and screening out, a very partial adverse de-selection of humankind – in say the insurance and employment sectors – with devastating consequences for the life chances of those individuals.

The decision-making about how and by whom research issues are defined, which methods are used, how projects are prioritised and funded when resources are limited are all relevant public health issues. For instance, a well researched drug may be able to reduce the health hazards presented by fatty, salty or sugary foods that other equally rigorous research has identified as leading to coronary heart diseases or diabetes. Pockets of such de-contextualised evidence may not inform good practice. Is the public health use of research findings to be one off-tactical options, as in prescribing such drugs, or is it to be strategic? To deal with a food industry that produces and aggressively targets and markets knowingly unhealthy foods made especially attractive to children, because of strong tastes/colours, creating eating habits that remain with them into adulthood? This is the burger and cola-lcohol culture. A strategic view would identify that some multi-national companies have activities in food production, processing and retailing which result in nurturing unhealthy dietary habits, which lead to later chronic and life threatening illnesses. These same companies may also research and supply the pharmaceutical products to treat such illnesses: a very profitable circle of activity but one that is a public health disaster. Again the tensions between upstream public health and downstream disease treatment and political reality of knowledge as power come strongly to the fore. Research on low nicotine tobacco products provides another example of business searching for ways to continue marketing hazardous products rather than ceasing to trade in goods dangerous to public health.

Health needs assessments and health impact assessments

All occupations look for useful, effective, practical, relevant, appropriate, cost-effective, affordable, time-saving tools to do their work. Health needs assessment is one such tool for the public health professional that has existed informally for centuries but has now been taken up by the Department of Health (DoH) for instance. It is not 'a quick fix' (Wright *et al.* 1998). The UK health policy requires local population plans to be drawn up and hence local health needs to be assessed. Public health professionals have been the source of most such assessments but of course these assessments, when based on standard epidemiological data, may well not accord with those of communities whose needs could be quite different to those identified by health professionals.

Advocates of health needs assessment highlight the fact that good health needs assessments will be systematic; draw on a range of methods including epidemiological, qualitative and comparative methods; identify needs 'that can benefit from health care or from wider social and environmental changes and be integrated into the 'planning and commissioning of local services'; be informed by what is required in terms of the process, resources and time (Wright *et al.* 1998: 1311).

Health needs assessment programmes have led some on to the critical area of health impact assessments (HIAs) with a recognition again that special tools are needed for particular products. There is no one HIA that will fit all requirements. The tools have been used to explore such topics as urban regeneration and transport. They require project screening, negotiation with key decision-makers, partnerships between interested parties including communities likely to be affected, a clear population and policy issue, systematic and timely approaches and appropriate evidence (SNAP 2000: 6).

Tools to address very specific aspects of public health have spun off from such programmes partly because of the powerful and early influence of environmental impact assessments (EIAs). Attempts have been made to produce environmental health impact tools (EHIAs) that draw on EIAs. This requires screening and scoping exercises to identify health hazards; agreed terms of reference and means to prepare impact assessments. This necessitates looking at community vulnerability and is then followed by an appraisal, negotiation and risk assessment on the proposed development and, where development occurs, future monitoring and surveillance of the problem (BMA 1998: 51). Effectively these are steps in a process rather than a tool and, as recent EIAs and EHIAs have shown with regard to dams in Turkey and India and waste disposal facilities in the United Kingdom, the results may be contested or interpreted in many ways.

Such tools may therefore be one of many that may be of use in public health. They are not suitable to every task and they may not work on any task.

Epidemiology

Epidemiology has been defined as:-

> The study of the distribution and determinants of health and disease related conditions in populations. It is concerned with both epidemic (excess of normal expectancy) and endemic (always present) conditions.... The basic premise of epidemiology is that disease is not randomly distributed across populations. (Shenker M in LaDou 1997)

This is viewed as the 'classical' quantitative public health tool. Whilst epidemiologists and public health professionals will be familiar with the difficulties and limitations of their methods and the problems of bias, confounders, population size, sample size, exposure measurement and so on, the public may not be. The public may become bemused by a series of seemingly contradictory public health studies on matters of real life interest to them. Alcohol is good/bad for you; contraceptives protect/damage your health, screening methods work/fail and so on. The result is that important public health messages may simply be ignored by the public who are now exposed, via the media, to confused and contradictory positions produced by public health research, but are not tutored in its limitations. The complexity and uncertainty of medical and scientific research is often underplayed by practitioners in the public arena and thus chaos or public anomie may result. These issues surrounding probabilistic and other risk assessments are addressed more fully in the environmental health chapter of this book.

A dearth of meaningful epidemiological study designs and data may present different but still major problems in informing effective public health practice. Which women smoke and why they continue to smoke, despite their awareness of the evidence of harm, is as important a question as how many. Similarly flawed epidemiological studies may warp, damage or destroy useful public health initiatives. This was seen with the study of survival of patients with breast cancer at the Bristol Self-Help Cancer Centre (Bagenal *et al.* 1990). Here the 'scientific' variables chosen for scrutiny did not adequately reflect the aims and aspirations – the type of evidence and assessment of good outcomes – of the women who had sought the intervention. This study has been described as 'bad research' and the way the research findings were broadcast in the media as 'extraordinarily inhumane' by other researchers (Stacey 1994: 93). It is as important in public health as in any other health field that ethical standards and responsibilities are interpreted broadly and hence research is guided by good ethical practice (Bradley and Burls 2000). This should automatically include respect for the participants' point of view.

Some have therefore questioned the funding of researchers and/or the shareholdings of researchers whose work relates to health matters associated with those companies with which they hold shares (Walker 2000). This is important in that the focus and methodologies of such research may potentially skew pharmaceutical, toxicological and even epidemiological evidence on public health problems and their proposed solutions. The whole question of medical and scientific fraud has been under-estimated and medical journals such as BMJ and Lancet are now making serious efforts to address the problem. Again these factors are important when critically appraising the research evidence.

Comprehensive epidemiological studies if done on a large enough scale, over a long period of time and with designs that minimise or make explicit potential bias have proved very effective ways of assessing disease causation in populations. This is, however, a very expensive process. It is also fundamentally limited because, although such studies may explore correlations between exposures and diseases, it will not necessarily identify important community contextual factors which may explain differences in individual disease patterns and immunities – or other potential public health risks or protectors which may inform disease prevention rather than causation alone. Whilst useful, narrow epidemiology effectively closes the stable door after the horse has bolted.

Toxicology and engineering are often portrayed as 'secure stables': we know that they are not. Technological optimists rely on the 'scientific method' and testing a null hypothesis usually derived from within their professional way of conceptualising issues. They may look for evidence that a process or product is hazardous within clear and calculated but nonetheless partial perceptions of what risks are. There may be an assumption that no hazard and no risk is present when data are lacking or incomplete. This is 'the prove it's dangerous' position. Similarly, studies may be produced that reveal 'positive' findings but they may be flawed and fail to provide a firm basis for public health policy making. Likewise studies may be conducted that are reported as 'negative' yet they may also be flawed. 'Negative' epidemiology – showing no effects on human health – may for instance be due to studies being too small to have statistically significant results; poorly designed and insensitive studies; invalid control groups; follow-up periods insufficient for effects to materialise or materialise fully or follow up incomplete; inaccurate exposure data; wrong exposure categories; exposures too low and/or too short to produce effects; too crude measures of morbidity; random errors and wrong or irrelevant morbidity indicators (Hernberg 1992). Hence, negative studies of potential pharmaceutical or environmental hazards have been claimed as proof of no risk when in fact there was an absence of good evidence to make that judgement rather than good evidence showing no such problem existed. Bovine Spongiform

Encephalopathy (BSE) and its role in variant Crentzfeldt Jakob disease (v-CJD) in human populations is a classic example.

The science of epidemiology, viewed as so critical to the development of 'academic', rigorous and high status public health medicine, has replaced clinical case studies as the most effective and credible method for identifying disease clusters. From this perspective clinical cases are viewed as statistically limited sources of information. However, non-epidemiological data linked to clinical cases or observations, have sometimes resulted in very effective actions. For instance the links between exposures to soot and cancer came from Percival Potts' clinical observations and case reports in the late eighteenth century. The links between exposure to vinyl chloride monomer and the rare liver cancer angiosarcoma came through primary care physicians near a US chemical plant connecting clinical cases. The 'Back to Sleep' campaign in the United Kingdom which cut 'sudden infant death' rates came from observational studies not conclusive physiological studies that could explain mechanisms of mortality (DoH 1998: 61).

Extensive epidemiological data may only provide a partial picture to some public health challenges and offer only partial or no solutions to problems. Epidemiology may for instance describe the distribution of teenage pregnancies and the health of the homeless but it offers less, and would not claim to, in terms of effective intervention strategies to address the problems so identified. Epidemiologists themselves have suggested that their discipline in its current form may have declining relevance to public health. Some suggest a molecular and social process approach to their subject linking technical and wider questions in what has been termed 'eco-epidemiology' (Wing 1994; Susser and Susser 1996a; Susser 1998).

Focus groups

'Focus Groups are fundamentally a way of listening to people and learning from them' (Morgan 1988: 9).

Focus groups were originally used in communication studies and market research to try to explore the effect of films and understand how customers think. More recently the methodology has been developed and increasingly used as a major tool in healthcare, public health and social research as a means of gaining insight into complex behaviours, such as perceptions of risk. The method has also come to represent a somewhat discredited activity among the public due to its political usage where claims are made that the findings from small, often less than rigorous group sessions are representative of public opinion or constitute a comprehensive public consultation exercise – a very useful tool for the party political 'spin doctor'. However, focus groups, as part of good research design, planned, executed, analysed and tested against accepted qualitative standards of rigour can produce useful and trustworthy evidence (Morgan 1988; Strauss and Corbin 1988).

Focus groups are semi-structured group sessions with participants purposively chosen for their shared experiences and drawn together to discuss specific broad areas of concern. Focus groups are overseen by a facilitator whose role is to guide wide ranging free discussion around a broad topic and to minimise any threats to validity of the data, such as dominant individuals or group conforming pressures, by encouraging equality of participation or probing and cross checking to clarify meaning. The explicit aim of this research approach is to capitalise on the interactive group process in order to explore how the participants themselves define and interpret their social realities. This approach has been deemed particularly useful for 'exploring people's knowledge and experiences and can be used to examine not only what people think but how they think and why they think that way' (Kitzinger 1996: 36). This knowledge can be readily utilised in public health policy and practice. Examples include exploration of teenagers' knowledge of, beliefs about and attitudes to contraception; understanding and behaviours associated with perceived risks of heart attacks; needs assessments informing programme developments for the elderly; exploration of the take-up of health education programmes for the self-management of asthma and children's road safety behaviours.

The group process utilises multiple forms of interactive communication which people use in everyday life such as humour, argument, body language, as they freely talk, question and exchange views between each other. These everyday dynamics are viewed as creating the possibilities for lay communication where 'knowledge and attitudes are not entirely encapsulated in reasoned responses to direct questions' (Kitzinger 1994: 109). In addition the method has been viewed as potentially non-discriminatory and empowering in that lack of language, technical or formal education does not exclude participation and the value of the shared experience validates those who feel they have nothing of value to say. For example, research with people with learning difficulties reveals the value of such approaches (Kitzinger 1996). The group situation is claimed to promote use of the participants' own vocabularies, language and interactive forms so revealing their thinking patterns, implicit cultural values, group norms and self-defined frameworks of relevance and priority. These dynamics can spontaneously take research into new dimensions, to areas which the professional researcher is unlikely to be in a position to conceptualise but which may be crucial to needs assessments or effective healthcare and public health practice.

For example, focus group work with the mothers of children with disabilities revealed differing lay/professional knowledge frameworks that are important to public health policy and practice. Here mothers employed socially, experientially, value-relevant ways of making sense of their worlds in contrast to professionals' more technical outcome focus (Watterson J 1999). This distinction goes beyond content and style of activity. It represents the expression of different conceptualisations, understandings and priorities permeating all aspects of experience of their children's healthcare. These different rationalities unwittingly contributed to discordant communications and understanding resulting in medical and neurodevelopmental therapy advice and interventions not being taken up. This focus group methodology did not just describe the difference (indeed the 'non-compliance' would not have been revealed as mothers reported telling therapists that they were carrying out therapy programmes when they were not) but it shed light onto the solution. In understanding the framework of mothers' own rationalities, professionals can both respect this and utilise it in practice. It is not just a matter of translating advice/changing the language of healthcare advice into a social remit but conceptualising the issues in a different way. Similarly, Kitzinger suggests that focus groups lend themselves to cross-cultural research work, including issues such as differential take up of health services or exploring differing risk behaviours within workplace cultures (Kitzinger 1996).

Focus groups present an effective means of gaining data of both breadth and depth in a relatively quick and cost-efficient way. However, there are practical difficulties relating to organising groups of appropriate size and composition in locations accessible to participants. Transcription and analysis of focus group data is complex and time consuming as the group is the unit of analysis with the sequencing of interactions critical to interpretation of the data and the identification of any threats to methodological validity such as conforming pressures producing group consensus. As discussed earlier in this chapter it is the conceptual/analytic themes which constitute the phenomena which are potentially transferable to other situations. For example, the differing value-relevant/outcome-task orientations of lay/professional interactions in childhood disability cited above is the analytic concept which is potentially transferable to other settings.

Confidentiality in the relatively public focus group setting poses further potential problems particularly as the group dynamics may encourage deep disclosures which participants may later regret. The moderator can promote high ethical standards by ensuring that ground rules for non-disclosure outside the group are set and observed. Health behaviours and experiences may be particularly sensitive areas and ethical research practice indicates that participants need to be empowered to withdraw and/or arrangements should be in place for follow-up support if required. For example, research may precipitate painful recall and in anticipation of this the researcher can build arrangements into the study for timely, qualified support, such as counselling, to be available (Watterson J 1999). However, these privacy and ethical considerations do not inhibit the use of focus groups for exploring sensitive public health issues. Indeed, Kitzinger argues that group dynamics help break down some taboos and cites work on bereavement, sexual violence, lovers of HIV positive people as examples of how the group setting offers a mutually supportive environment in which mutual trust can develop and fundamental disclosures such as the real reasons why known public health messages may not be taken up by their target groups (Kitzinger 1996).

Hence, focus groups provide a useful research tool to generate information and insights relevant to communities and the public understanding of health and health behaviours. Some of the costs/benefits have been outlined but perhaps their greatest strength is the specific use and privileging of lay communications and conceptualisations to inform effective public health policy and practice.

Participatory research

This could include such methods as rapid appraisal, community, lay and worker epidemiology and citizens' juries. The classic qualitative tools in public health outside the northern hemisphere may also rely on verbal autopsies where interviews with family and community contacts of someone who has died may provide additional morbidity and mortality data linked to public health threats to health. Indian and Asian groups have used these techniques quite successfully to address a wide range of often hitherto neglected public health problems relating to gender, rural communities and access to public health services (De Koning and Martin 1996).

Risk assessment, management and communication

These methods are discussed in the chapter on environmental health. The assumptions in terms of public health presentations may be that at one level risks can be quantified relatively easily and the public simply do not understand those risks. From this scenario it follows that this must then necessitate better risk education for the public. However, if public perceptions are one of the starting points for public health, the solutions must then necessitate the education of scientists in the different but not inferior risk assessment understanding of the public and the often different but not inferior risk management perceptions of the public which may not have been prioritised. Yet, it is exactly this area that needs to be addressed if public health practice is to be effective. Acknowledging, understanding and respecting that there are differing perceptions of reality and differing types of legitimate evidence highlight the differing but often complementary approaches to evidence-based public health practice that this chapter seeks to explore.

Conventional participatory research operates in the context of 'lay/worker/community' activity for the collective public health good. In the work environment this approach has a part to play in the process of vetting substances, processes, materials, buildings, factories and other types of plant and installations. In the past we have witnessed a global overconfidence by scientists, regulators and politicians when dealing with potential public health risks and problems. Their inability to deal with uncertainty, their failure to take data gaps seriously when carrying out risk assessments, their failure to go beyond very narrow risk assessments and skewed cost–benefit analyses which constantly favour capital over community and workers is sadly obvious. The failure to recognise, research or act on research – when potential problems were flagged – with BSE, asbestos, Diethylstilbestrol (DES) and other endocrine disrupters illustrates the large scale and the major consequences of such over-confidence or sometimes failure of courage to tackle powerful commercial interests.

Daily some communities and some continents live with the consequences of the failure of such narrow approaches – whether in Clydebank from asbestos-related diseases, Bhopal from pesticide manufacture failures, the Ukraine from the Chernobyl disaster, Russia with TB, Africa with HIV. Lay/worker/community action on public health issues can highlight these failures and bring important precautionary approaches to effectively bear on decision-making as well as inform solutions and the factors which might facilitate or inhibit the application of such new knowledge.

In the United Kingdom, groups of women in Boston, Lincolnshire and the Women's Environment Network (WEN) breast cancer survey, involved with mapping hazards and risks in communities in partnership with local people, illustrate how communities themselves, sometimes supported by NGOs, can explore possible health issues and ways to promote health (WEN 1999). For several years the United Kingdom has been top of the world league for deaths from breast cancer in women. Local community groups concerned about the high incidence of breast cancer in their areas have often met resistance and apathy from public health professionals. The WEN women themselves organised a variety of means to investigate hitherto neglected aspects of the possible aetiology of breast cancer – through risk mapping and pollution plotting exercises in their communities.

Their aim was to raise awareness of the lack of activity on primary prevention of the disease and the fact that perhaps at best only 40 per cent of all breast cancer cases have established causes.

They asked what role environmental factors could play in the disease and why so little data were available about environmental exposures and environmental risks related to breast cancer. The WEN breast cancer project has provided a community-based means for such issues to be explored which may complement or possibly question some of the conventional tools used by epidemiologists. WEN and other NGOs represent the prudent decision-makers, and advocates of the precautionary principle in the public health field. Again, drawing on the theme of this chapter in presenting the case for acknowledging a variety of evidences, this participatory research is one aspect, of what can become a polarised picture, of strategies informed by partnerships of evidence that are required to tackle public health risks.

These 'participatory' studies have also used well-established and new traditional research methods such as Geographical Information Systems (GIS) but their roots lie in the risk mapping activities of workers in a Fiat plant in Italy many years ago. The maps so prepared rely on worker/community knowledge of processes and procedures rather than managerial and 'expert' assessments which may reflect theoretical evidence rather than the real practice of processes and chemical usage. Again, differing public health theories underpin differing approaches to risk and to epidemiology. Prudent decision-makers, referred to in Chapter 1, who use lay epidemiology approaches are searching for public health data to demonstrate that there are no major risks associated with hazards: the burden of proof lies with the manufacturer/government to show processes are 'safe'. In contrast to the expert hierarchical view of evidence, this approach is informed but not dictated by science and scientific methods and recognises both the value and the limits of our scientific knowledge.

Gaining more comprehensive evidence entails opening up the research process to ensure communities and workers can contribute to and influence any changes proposed as a result of the research undertaken. However, this strategy carries potential political and economic costs for business.

The benefits of participatory research can be considerable. For instance, such research may play a role in exposing unrecognised levels of disease or through studying subjective symptoms in an effective way. This is the case with regard to Myalgic Encephalomyelitis (ME) or Chronic Fatigue Syndrome (CFS) where there has recently been medical recognition of the existence of a disease previously rejected as such by medicine. More controversy surrounds multiple chemical sensitivity (MCS), syndromes, work-related upper limb disorders and repetitive strain injuries, asthma aetiology and occupational stress and all are now being explored by participatory research. These methods may be cost-effective or low-cost ways of identifying a wide range of exposures to possible disease causes and outcomes through interactive approaches. They are able to deal with rapidly changing situations and almost automatically they increase the capacity of communities and workers to involve themselves in public health. This is because the methods recognise and use knowledge and experience of communities in identifying particular health risks. Such methods also help to inform solutions and provide new approaches to conceptualising knowledge, enhancing the potential for action outcomes from research findings. Finally, they raise awareness of policy makers linked to an identification of key local concerns (Loewenson *et al.* 1995; Loewenson 1999).

There are of course weaknesses attached to participatory research. For instance the assumption that there is an identifiable community perspective is problematic and this may mean that no precise quantification of a particular problem can be identified. There could be inaccurate or incomplete or partial perspectives provided on an issue bearing in mind that there is a major difference between lay perceptions and lay epidemiology. Lay perceptions of public health problems could include misconceptions about the nature, causes and prevention of disease such as coronary heart disease. This has been widely discussed but no lay epidemiology studies of such diseases have been undertaken which might shed some light on the confusing messages, presented via media reports to the public, of epidemiologists professional understanding of a variety of diseases. Similarly lay perceptions of the causes of malaria in West Africa have been linked to eating unripened fruit. Again no lay epidemiology studies of the disease have apparently been conducted and there may or may not be an association between malaria and these observations of the public.

Rapid appraisal

This is an approach which encapsulates a major strand of public health encompassing the tools of health needs assessment and health impact assessments. 'Rapid appraisal is primarily a methodology which provides timely, relevant information for decision-makers on the pressing issues they face in project and programme settings (Kumar 1994 cited by Ong 1996: 3). Hence, it can be a diagnostic tool, an agent for change or both. It does not necessarily draw on communities in the appraisal as lay epidemiology always would. The method proposes that communities, whether geographic or workplace-based, should be recognised as public health decision-makers as well as the politicians and scientists. The methods that rapid appraisals deploy are very familiar to those engaged in lay epidemiology. They might include any or a mixture of the following: mapping matrices that are also discussed in the occupational health chapter, focus groups that are discussed elsewhere in this chapter, time lines and trend analysis. The approach is often semi-structured, multi-disciplinary, flexible and innovative. It may be faster than 'conventional methods'. There is a field work emphasis to the approach and a reliance on learning directly from local people. It focuses on 'insights, hypotheses, best bets rather than final truths or fixed recommendations' (Ong 1996: 2).

Key steps in the process could include clearly defining the purpose of the appraisal and identifying target groups and agencies. This would be followed by identifying a leader or team to conduct rapid appraisal and organising participatory workshops. Fieldwork and observation would develop with secondary data collection, interviews and analysis of the data. These data bases would inform the prioritisation of needs. Crucially there would be feed back of findings to the community and discussions of proposed actions leading to the development of a programme of change. Evaluation of the work and, if necessary, redefinition of priorities might be identified with the need to explore the possibility of a second rapid appraisal or future action based on the first appraisal (Ong 1996: 9).

Lay epidemiology

Lay epidemiology is 'the process by which lay persons gather statistics and other information and also direct and marshal the knowledge and resources of experts in order to understand the epidemiology of diseases' (Brown 1989).

In the 1920s and 1930s the physician Sir Thomas Legge who was an early user of 'sentinel' events to trigger investigations of health hazards, (Legge 1934: 25–9). He used observational data from workers to identify hitherto relatively unknown risks. For instance, he visited a docks site where the dockers themselves had linked work with a hard wood to cases of ill-health in their members when no physician had done so.

Lay epidemiology should be a major strand of participatory research. However, it is often neglected as it sometimes appears difficult to implement and perhaps more importantly may be perceived as de-valued and open to challenge by those professional regulators and scientists committed to concepts of methodologically hierarchical evidence rather than differing evidences being informed by differing values, criteria of rigour and usefulness. Lay epidemiology might draw on qualitative and quantitative research methods in order to generate comprehensive, rich data. The uses of the technique are many and varied and do not simply relate to the investigation of a health hazard or to confirm or disconfirm scientific evidence about correlations and causes of diseases. They also contain important community, individual, political and social elements (Watterson 1994, Popay and Williams 1994, 1996).

Lay epidemiology may inform communities about public health problems and solutions. By involving communities in public health policy and the monitoring of practical policy implementation, lay epidemiology has the potential to sustain and empower communities and individuals in an organisational and possibly social context. The approach also has potential to help change attitudes to disease causation, disease prevention and the effectiveness of public health measures. In addition it may possibly serve to educate professionals, through lay groups, about new or different public health perspectives. It is part of a campaign for positive change.

Lay epidemiology studies can include tools, mechanisms, techniques and methods that appear 'easy' but are not and may be complex in terms of data gathering. Different types of data are generated and used differently. Studies may generate similar data to that used by epidemiologists and toxicologists but often this is not the case and they could be more comprehensive, experiential, up to date, relevant, better informed. They can be qualitative – records and histories may provide supporting information in conventional epidemiology whereas here it represents core data.

Quantitative methodological concerns regarding the rigour of research including validity of recall, reliability and verifiability, issues about location and length of exposure and exposure levels in conventional epidemiology are shared with lay methods. However, records of incidents, accounts of exposures, details of suspected adverse effects may all be more richly documented in lay epidemiology with the participants' perceived experience acknowledged as their reality unlike other sorts of epidemiological study.

Data collection in lay, community and worker studies may also be presented in forms readily recognised and accepted by conventional epidemiologists. These approaches are illustrated, to some extent, by the conventional but imaginative Indonesian pesticide studies carried out recently on behalf of the FAO by Helen Murphy and her colleagues (1998). These methods include recruiting local health workers and key community activists to gather data through observation and interviews; using house, locality and body maps and also questionnaires comprehensible and quickly understood by the local population in which the study was being conducted. Such methods would not necessarily be familiar to those conducting traditional 'field epidemiology' (Gregg 1996).

Lay epidemiology is relatively cheap to do, draws on local data, can utilise people pooling knowledge encompassing a socio-participative/participative model. It nurtures transparency in study design, execution and analysis and in this context it is an open process that is inclusive, potentially empowering and recognises uncertainty. It is a positive process which will usually create many benefits with the potential to go beyond the rhetoric of transparency and empowerment as it is embedded in community practice.

Lay epidemiology complements and may triangulate with other methods and reflects current international and national agendas relating to WHO Charter on Environment in promoting the involvement of local communities in their health care. It may help to facilitate actions to address health inequalities and unlike conventional studies may provide early warning of problems before disasters occur. It has been associated with linking worker and geographical communities as the environmental justice campaign of Friends of the Earth in Scotland has done in bringing trade unions, communities and environmentalists together to investigate public health issues.

Lay epidemiology may focus on small groups and the evidence does not lend itself to traditional concepts of sample population generalisability but can offer the analytical generalisability of concepts and insights of qualitative paradigms. Yet, small studies may produce quite original and important data which can provide real benefits in terms solving problems, engaging communities and creating structures through which wider public health debates and policy formulation can be conducted. As with conventional epidemiology there are perennial problems of identifying random/ causal clusters. Health professionals may resist and sometimes oppose any discussion of the issues raised and there may be a lack of good data on exposures although communities can produce experiential evidence about the reality of exposures rather than assumed projections.

The interface between conventional and lay epidemiology Some potential problems inherent in lay epidemiology, in addition to the methodological issues discussed above, include access to resources which may relate to challenges to the credibility of the method if viewed as insufficiently rigorous by professional scientists relying on positivist concepts of evidence. According to the epidemiologist Sven Hernberg 'the prevailing view' is usually subjective in science' (Hernberg 1992). Therefore when epidemiology produces results that are inconclusive, then lively debates ensues. The terrain will often be hotly contested by both scientists and the public. Only when many and usually large studies have been produced can assessments be made with some certainty and the reliance now on meta analyses – reviewing all the studies in a field – is considerable. However, epidemiology is only of value after exposures have occurred, either in prospective or retrospective studies It can be very expensive and time-consuming to do elaborate studies which, at the end of the day, will produce information about circumscribed associations and correlations rather than demonstrate how and why causation did, did not occur within populations. As public health is concerned with populations, epidemiological work has been critical to understanding the risks of such threats as exposure to tobacco, radiation, air pollution and so on. Such data have been appropriately produced and strong enough to inform effective public health policy making at this wider level.

Lay epidemiology has the potential to produce knowledge that meets the needs of communities and NGOs whose priorities may be quite different to those of the established scientific community.

Table 2.1   Types of lay epidemiology

1. Epidemiologists design, carry out, analyse and present the study.
2. Epidemiologists design, study and train and use lay staff to carry out survey. Epidemiologists analyse and present data.
3. Epidemiologists invite lay people to contribute to design of study protocol. Lay staff carry out questionnaire surveys, interviews. Epidemiologists analyse, present data.
4. Epidemiologists invite lay people to contribute to study design. Lay people carry out surveys. Epidemiologists, with lay people, analyse and present results.
5. Lay people identify problem and invite epidemiologists to investigate the problem. Back to (1).
6. Lay people identify problems, involve epidemiologists. Joint protocol is drawn up. Back to (3) and (4).
7. Lay people identify problem, involve epidemiologists. Joint protocol. Lay people and epidemiologists jointly investigate problem, analyse results. Joint presentation of results.

Source: Watterson AE 1999; Watterson AE 2000.

For instance operationalisation of the precautionary principle often requires information about data gaps rather than 'data rich' but 'information poor' masses of statistical/epidemiological data.

Lay epidemiology may or may not be totally excluded from conventional epidemiological studies. A continuum of both approaches ranging from solely conventional to research controlled, conducted and delivered by lay groups is set out in Table 2.1. In most instances, the type of lay epidemiology studies that have been conducted fall into categories 2–5.

The benefits of lay, worker and community-led health studies

Lay studies may use a range of traditional and innovative methods. In keeping with the theme of this chapter, the advantages of a pragmatic, problem solving approach to knowledge production by using methods eclectically in order to reach groups, populations, problems and issues that conventional methods alone are not equipped to deal with is advocated. The question then is 'how can they be introduced more widely and supported more clearly? The process may be helped by:

- strengthening the means available for social, economic or geographical communities to participate and indeed initiate lay/community epidemiology;
- ensuring that 'no cost' freedom of information about disease and prevention is available at community level and ensuring easy access to such information;
- creating information systems that disseminate information rather than restrict information because communities do not know what information is available or are only given information if they ask very specific questions;
- re-educating health workers in community epidemiology principles and techniques;
- incorporating the principle of communities in the monitoring, review and audit of public health hazards into the new training of health and technical staff in public and private sectors;
- involving all regional health authorities, trusts, local authorities, commercial bodies adopting the WHO Charter on Environment and Health with a commitment to implement its principles and practice. Public Health Medicine Departments in health authorities around the country should have a key role in this process as should community health councils;
- central and local government and other funding agencies ensuring that lay/community epidemiology is built in as a requirement for any research grants or programmes which involve working on communities or health hazards affecting particular groups.

Conclusion

In summary, there are various tools available to public health practitioners and communities in the search for the types of evidence that will help them to address often complex concerns at global, national and local levels. The choice of topics to be studied and the tools to be used are not value free and so the technical use of the tools must be linked to awareness of their origins, development, application and impact.

The next chapter will examine international influences on public health primarily through economic drivers.

References

Ashton J (ed.) (1994) *The Epidemiological Imagination.* Open University Press, Buckingham.

Ashton J (1999) 'Past and Present Public Health in Liverpool' in Griffiths and Hunter (eds) *Perspectives in Public Health.* Radcliffe Medical Press, Abingdon, pp 23–323.

Atkin K, Lunt N and Thompson C (ed.) (1999) *Evaluating Community Nursing.* Bailliere Tindall, Edinburgh.

Bagenal FS, Easton DF, Harris E and Chilvers CED (1990) Survival of patients with breast cancer attending Bristol Cancer Self Help Centre. *Lancet* **336**: 606–610.

BMA (1998) *Health and Environmental Impact Assessments.* Earthscan, London.

Bradley P and Burls A (eds) (2000) *Ethics in Public and Community Health.* Routledge, London.

Brown P (ed.) (1989) *Perspectives in Medical Sociology.* Belmont CA, Wadsworth.

Burls A and Cabello-Lopez J (2000) 'Research methods in health' in Bradley and Burls (eds) *Ethics in Public and Community Health.* Routledge, London, pp 135–47.

Bury T and Mead J (1998) *Evidence-based Healthcare: A Practical Guide for Therapists.* Butterworth Heinemann, Oxford.

Carter Y, Shaw S and Thomas C (1999) *An Introduction to Qualitative Methods for Health Professionals.* Royal College of General Practitioners, London.

Cuff EC, Sharrock W and Francis DW (1990) *Perspectives in Sociology.* 3rd edn. Routledge, London.

Dawes M, Davies P, Gray A, Mant J, Seers K and Snowball R (1999) *Evidence-based Practice: A Primer for Health Care Professionals.* Churchill Livingstone, Edinburgh.

Davey Smith G and Ebrahim S (2001) Epidemiology – is it time to call it a day? *Int J Epidemiol* **30**(1): 1–11.

De Koning K and Martin M (1996) *Participatory Research in Health: Issues and Experiences.* Zed Books, London.

Department of Health (1998) *Quantification of the Effects of Air Pollution on Health in the United Kingdom.* Committee on the Medical effects of Air Pollutants. HMSO, London.

Gregg MB (1996) *Field Epidemiology.* Oxford University Press, New York.

Griffiths S and Hunter D (1999) *Perspectives in Public Health.* Radcliffe Medical Press, Abingdon.

Hernberg S (1992) *Introduction to Occupational Epidemiology.* Lewis Publishers, Chelsea, Michigan.

Jenkinson C (ed.) (1997) *Assessment and Evaluation of Health and Medical Care.* Open University Press, Buckingham.

Kitzinger J (1994) The methodology of focus groups: the importance of interaction between research participants. *Sociol Health Illness* **16**(1): 103–21.

Kitzinger J (1996) 'Introducing focus groups' in Mays N and Pope C (eds) *Qualitative Research in Healthcare.* British Medical Journal Publishing, London, pp 36–45.

Loader BD (1999) 'Informational health networks: health care organisation in the information age' in Purdy P and Banks M (eds) *Health and Exclusion: Policy and Practice in Health provision.* Routledge, London and New York, pp 179–99.

La Dou J (ed.) (1997) *Occupational and Environmental Medicine.* Appleton Lange, Connecticut.

Legge TM (1934) *Industrial Maladies.* Oxford University Press, Oxford.

Loewenson R, Biocca M, Laurell AC and Hogstedt C (1995) Participatory approaches in occupational health research: a review. *Med Lav* **86**(3): 263–71.

Loewenson R (1999) People centred science and globalisation: putting the public back into public health policy. *Int J Occup Environ Health* **5**(1) 65–71.

Morgan DL (1988) *Focus Groups and Qualitative Research.* Sage, Thousand Oaks, California.

Muir Gray JA (1997) *Evidence-based Healthcare.* Churchill Livingstone, Edinburgh.

Murphy E, Dingwall R, Greatbatch D, Parker S and Watson P (1998) Qualitative research methods in health technology assessment: a review of the literature. *Health Technol Assess* **2**(16): 1–276.

Ong BN and Humphris G (1994) 'Prioritising needs with communities: rapid appraisal methodologies in health' in Popay and Williams (eds) *Researching the People's Health.* Routledge, London, pp 58–84.

Ong BN (1996) *Rapid Appraisal and Health Policy.* Chapman and Hall, London.

Popay J and Williams G (eds) (1994) *Researching the People's Health.* Routledge, London.

Popay J and Williams G (1996) Public health research and lay knowledge. *Soc Sc Med* **42**: 759–68.

Popper K (1959) *The Logic of Scientific Discovery.* Hutchinson.

Purdy P and Banks M (eds) (1999) *Health and Exclusion: Policy and Practice in Health Provision.* Routledge, London and New York.

Rice C, Roberts H, Smith SJ and Bryce C (1994) 'Its like teaching your child to swim in a pool full of alligators – lay voices and professional research on child accidents' in Popay J and Williams G (eds) *Researching the People's Health.* Routledge, London, pp 115–33.

Rosen G (1974) *From Medical Police to Social Medicine.* Science History Publications, New York.

Scottish Needs Assessment Programme [SNAP] (2000) *Health Impact Assessment: Piloting the Process in Scotland.* SNAP, Glasgow.

Stacey M (1994) 'The Power of lay knowledge' in Popay J and Williams G (eds) *Researching the People's Health.* Routledge, London, pp 85–98.

Strauss A and Corbin J (1998) *Basics of Qualitative Research.* Sage, Thousand Oaks, California.

Susser M and Susser E (1996a) Choosing a future for epidemiology 1. Eras and paradigms. *Am J Public Health* **86**(5): 668–73.

Susser M and Susser E (1996b) Choosing a future for epidemiology 11. From black box to Chinese boxes and eco-epidemiology. *Am J Public Health* **86**(5): 674–7.

Susser M (1998) Does risk factor epidemiology put epidemiology at risk? Peering into the future. *J Epidemiol Community Health* **52**(10): 608–11.

Walker M (2000) Your money and your life: Britain's cancer charities. *The Ecologist.* 2 November, p 6.

Watterson AE (1994). Whither lay epidemiology in occupational and environmental health? *J Public Health Med* **16**: 270–4.

Watterson AE (1999) Why epidemiologists may fail worker and community groups and what can be done about it. London School of Hygiene and Tropical Medicine.

Watterson AE (2000) Lay, community and worker 'epidemiology': an integrating strand in participatory research. *No more Bhopals*, Sambhvanba Clinic, Bhopal, India.

Watterson J (1999) 'An exploratory study of mothers' views and experiences of providing practical care for their children with delayed motor development'. Unpublished MA thesis, De Montfort University, Leicester.

Wing S (1994) Limits of epidemiology. *Med Global Surv* **1**: 74–86.

Wright J, Williams R and Wilkinson JR (1998) Health needs assessment: development and importance of health needs assessment. *BMJ* **316**: 1310–13.

Women's Environmental Network (1999) *Putting Breast Cancer on the Map.* 87 Worship St. London EC2A 2BE, UK.

3

International Influences on Public Health

Julie Prowse

Introduction

'The last one hundred years have seen a greater improvement in health than at any time in the last three millennia' (WHO 2000: 4). The evidence shows that not all countries or individuals have benefited equally, the poorest 20 per cent of people in the world are approximately ten times more likely to die before the age of 14 than the richest 20 per cent, whilst more than 90 per cent of maternal and child deaths occur in developing countries (DFID 2000a: 8, 2000b).

This chapter examines the key issues that affect public health at a macro level by analysing the policies and interventions of global institutions such as the World Bank, International Monetary Fund (IMF) and World Trade Organisation (WTO). At a micro level the effects of these organisations on public health are explored in particular chapters elsewhere in the book. The first section presents an overview of global institutions such as the World Bank, IMF and WTO and the factors that shaped them. The next section examines the strategies of the IMF and World Bank and the effects on developing countries by analysing the impact of debt and debt reduction policies on public health. Current measures being implemented such as the Heavily Indebted Poor Countries Initiative and the Poverty Reduction Growth Facility are reviewed. The conclusion explores the issue of globalisation and the implications for international organisations and public health.

Public health practitioners themselves nationally and internationally are clearly directly influenced in what they can and can not do by these political-economic factors. Most importantly global and national economic issues will determine food and water supplies, housing numbers and standards, sustainability, income and poverty, transport, climate – the macro public health influences – in every country in the world. Such economic factors will also directly determine the budgets of public health workers, their pharmaceutical budgets, their education and training programmes, staff levels and other resources. So one of vital skills required of the public health practitioner is the ability to lobby for change or at least contribute to the lobbying of others on the global stage with regard to globalisation and economic growth. This 'economic' element is a theme that runs through all the chapters of the book and is covered explicitly especially in the practice of the public health physician (Chapter 4), the housing specialist (Chapter 7), the environmental health officer (Chapter 8) and the occupational health and safety practitioner (Chapter 9).

Development policies have been widely recognised for some time as impacting upon health through the factors described in this chapter (Cooper Weil *et al.* 1990). Trade, agriculture, industry, energy policies, housing and related planning matters all feed into, reflect or are damaged by development policies. The consequences of poor development policies for public health has been neglected. This chapter explores some of those deficiencies and the bigger picture.

Non-government Agencies (NGOs) such as Oxfam, Save the Children and Medecins Sans Frontieres although not covered extensively in this chapter, play an important part in developing countries. The role of these agencies has changed since their inception with the type of interventions and policies pursued determined by recipient countries rather than NGOs (Turner 2001; Beattie 2001a). Increasingly projects that involve NGOs are managed by development agencies local to the country or region. Consultants from NGOs may be used for specific projects such as water and sanction, public health assessment and promotion, nutrition and food security, logistics, project management programme coordinator, accountancy and office management, but it is local workers that are used to deliver projects. NGOs play a vital role in bringing international attention to issues such as global poverty and providing critical comment on the policies of the IMF, World Bank and WTO. The involvement of NGOs in campaigns such as 'Trade not Aid' 'Drop the Debt' and 'Jubilee 2000' has resulted in alliances between NGOs and other organisations that target the policies of global institutions and raised the profile of world poverty and debt (Peel 2001).

Factors that influence public health

Some of the factors that influence public health and are used to make cross-national comparisons relate directly to primary care. The WHO (WHO/UNICEF 1978: 3) define primary health care (PHC) as:

> primary health care forms an integral part of a country's development and health system. It is the first level of contact for the individual, family and community with the health system, bringing health care as close as possible to where people live and work, and constitutes the first element of a continuing health care process.

PHC was intended to cover the following key areas:

• health education
• food supply and nutrition
• water and sanitation
• maternal and child health
• immunisation
• prevention and control of locally endemic diseases
• treatment of common diseases and injuries
• provision of essential drugs.

These PHC areas are invaluable for comparing and assessing the level of public health in a country and in Chapter 6, the United Kingdom weighting and implementation of these areas will be discussed in depth. The extent to which these measures can be achieved globally is determined by a number of factors.

The wealth of a nation is one of the key indicators of health status. The World Bank (2000a: 335) classifies the economy of a country on the basis of Gross National Product (GNP) per capita as either low income $755 or less per year; lower-middle income, $756–$2995; upper-middle income, $2996–9265; and high income $9266 or more. France (7.7 per cent), Germany (8.8 per cent), United States (6.6 per cent) and the United Kingdom (5.7 per cent) are classified as high income countries and spend a greater proportion of Gross Domestic Product (GDP) on health, than low income nations such as Nigeria (0.2 per cent) and Georgia (0.7 per cent) (World Bank 2001a). Although these criteria are useful a country may be classified as high income but still have a significant proportion of the population living in poverty and unable to access health care, due to income disparities or the cost of health care (Field 1989; George and Taylor-Gooby 1996; Wall 1996).

A range of measures demonstrate the irrevocable link between the wealth and poverty of an individual and the effects on public health. The Human Poverty Index (HPI) measures deprivation by examining five aspects that provide evidence of the level of public health and indicate where resources need to be invested. The HPI index covers:

- Poverty
- Illiteracy
- Malnutrition amongst children
- Early death
- Poor health care
- Poor access to safe water.

The significance of these indicators can be illustrated by examining access to clean water. This measure provides evidence of whether a country's general level of public health is improving or deteriorating. Data collected between 1982 and 1995 revealed that in France, United Kingdom and Germany, nearly 100 per cent of the population had access to safe water. Substantial improvements have been achieved in Cote d'Ivoire and Ethiopia where only 20 per cent and 4 per cent accessed clean water in 1982, but by 1995 this figure had risen to 72 per cent and 26 per cent respectively. During the same period there was a decline in the proportion of people accessing safe water in Albania and the Zambia (World Bank 2000a). The data collected for these countries, based on the HPI index, demonstrates a correlation between all the areas and the level of public health provided.

The political stability of a country and the level of corruption is another factor that determines the health status of a population. Nations that have been involved in sustained conflicts such as Rwanda, the former Yugoslavia, Afghanistan and Sierra Leone devote fewer resources to public health. Conflict may be a major reason for poverty in many countries as funding that should have been invested in food production or public health is used to uphold corrupt regimes or maintain a war (Red Cross 1996). The devastating effects of conflict also undermines disease prevention and immunisation. One of the targets set by the WHO (2000) was the global eradication of polio by 2002. This has virtually been achieved in India, where reports of polio have declined following a mass immunisation programme (Pilling 2001). Angola, Afghanistan, Democratic Republic of Congo, Somalia and Sudan still report polio where immunisations programmes are almost impossible to provide because of continued conflict. The problems that chronic mismanagement, political corruption and crop failure can cause is illustrated by the plight of Malawi. A country that could produce sufficient food to sustain its citizens, Malawi, is facing a food crisis that is estimated to affect seven of the ten million population as the nation faces imminent famine (Turner 2002).

In addition to the factors influencing public health discussed in Chapter 1, the policies and strategies of international organisations play a vital role in determining public health and will be evaluated next.

Economic factors

The need to ensure global economic growth and the stability of nations has been the impetus for the creation of a range of international agencies that include the World Bank, the IMF and the WTO. During the 1920s and 1930s a series of economic cycles of 'booms and busts' occurred, that resulted in the collapse of international trade markets, the devaluation of currencies and mass unemployment (Curwen 1997; Griffiths and Wall 1999). To address these problem many countries, particularly the United States, adopted 'trade protectionist policies' designed to protect their markets by restricting the import of goods and imposing tariffs (Curwen 1997). The effect of this action was a global recession, the collapse of international economic stability and had a profound adverse effect on public health.

The Second World War brought the depression to a close but, in order to avoid a repetition of the 1930s, many nations were determined to create a number of international organisations that would manage and police global issues like trade, finance, health and security (Parkin *et al.* 2000). From 1942 onwards a series of meetings were held in the United States to determine how the post-war period was to be managed (George and Sabelli 1994). The result of these endeavours was the creation in 1944 of the Bretton Woods Institutions, which comprised of the World Bank and the IMF. The founders believed these global institutions would ensure a better post-war society based on financial growth and reduce the risk of further conflict. However, these organisations were conceived not only as economic but also as political institutions designed to ensure future stability and prosperity. In pursuing these aims both the World Bank and the IMF have been accused of not being politically neutral and implementing policies that have benefited developed G7 nations (United Kingdom, France, United States, Canada, Italy, Japan and Germany) and detrimentally affected developing countries. The evidence suggests that despite the intervention of a range of agencies during the last fifty years the populations of developing countries continue to suffer from preventable diseases, and to be unacceptably exposed to a number of health and environmental problems (Vaughan *et al.* 1996; Ehiri and Prowse 1999).

The Bretton Woods Institutions

The World Bank

The World Bank is both a bank and a development institution which provides loans to low and lower-middle income countries. In contrast, the IMF focuses on short-term macroeconomic policy, maintains a surveillance of world economies and provides technical and financial assistance in the form of concessional and non-concessional loans.

The World Bank contains five agencies that undertake a variety of roles, reflecting their areas of responsibility and policy.

The International Bank for Reconstruction and Development (IBRD) and the International Development Association (IDA) provide development loans and assistance to developing countries. The International Finance Corporation (IFC), Multilateral Investment Guarantee Agency (MIGA) and International Centre for Settlement of Investment Disputes (ICSID) are mainly concerned with promoting private sector investment in developing countries (George 1992; World Bank 2000b). The World Bank key activities are defined as:

- Investing in people, particularly thorough basic health and education
- Focusing on social development, inclusion, governance and institution building as key elements of poverty reduction
- Strengthening the ability of a government to deliver quality services, efficiently and transparently
- Protecting the environment
- Supporting and encouraging private business development
- Promoting reforms to create a stable macroeconomic environment, conducive to investment and long term planning (World Bank 2000b: 1).

The IBRD was created in 1944 to provide loans to European nations for post-war reconstruction. In 1948, the bank expanded its role and offered 'Project Loans' to assist developing countries to finance specific developments such as dams, roads, hydration, and electricity. Strategic projects in education, agriculture and health concentrated on literacy, vaccinations and increasing crop production (George and Sabelli 1994). Finance for the IBRD comes from the issue and selling of bonds to investors and the provision of debt securities. The World Bank only negotiates with governments, not individuals and the money borrowed, unlike aid, has to be repaid. The repayment of a loan is spread over a 15–20-year period, with no payment required for the first five years. The IBRD never cancels a loan, the debt is rescheduled, but countries must pay the interest, calculated at the current rate (George 1992; Branford and Kucinski 1990). Countries who borrow from the IBRD are low or middle-income countries such as China, India, Hungary, Poland and Turkey. Due to the immense power the World Bank exerts over public and private sources of capital, countries always repay loans first and this takes precedence over social programmes such as health and education (Chossudovsky 1997; Oxfam 1996). As a result of sustained poverty 3 billion people live on less than $2 a day, 40 000 die of preventable disease every day and 1.3 billion still do not have access to clean drinking water (World Bank 2000b).

The second key area of activity for the World Bank is the IDA established in 1960 to provide concessional assistance in the form of soft loans called 'credits' to the world's poorest countries. These nations are unable to afford IBRD rates or secure finance from other sources. In order to qualify for IDA assistance a country must have a per capita income of less than $885 a year and a successful track record in managing development projects (World Bank 2001b). Normally, the IDA lends $4 billion a year for projects that include primary education, basic health services, clean water and sanitation (World Bank 2000b). Currently, 2.3 billion people from 78 countries are eligible for loans from the IDA who lent $5.177 billion to the following areas in 2000 (World Bank 2000b: 2):

- Africa – lending was increased to those countries demonstrating good or improving performance and included; Madagascar, Senegal, Uganda and Zambia. The IDA made a substantial loan to Rwanda to assist in maintaining stability following the genocide of 1994.
- Asia, China and India – received funding to support poverty reduction. Indonesia received funding to support development following the fiscal crisis of 1998.
- Europe and Central Asia – lending supported projects that assisted reconstruction and transition management in Albania, Armenia and Georgia. Countries emerging from civic conflict such as Bosnia and Herzegovina also received funding.

The funding for the IDA comes from governments or donors, predominately G7, countries who pledge amounts (World Bank 2000c). Loans made by the IDA, differ from the IBRD in that they are virtually interest free and repayment is over a 35–40-year period. No payment is required for the first ten years, however borrowers pay a 1 per cent fee to cover the cost of administration (George and Sabelli 1994). IDA loans must be repaid which has meant that a significant proportion of developing countries are in debt to both the World Bank and the IMF with major public health implications.

During 2000, the World Bank lent a total of $15.3 billion (World Bank 2000c) with Latin America and the Caribbean receiving just over $4 billion and Eastern Europe and Central Asia, $2979 billion. The key projects financed were Public Sector Management change (14.8 per cent), Financial Sector Development (12 per cent) and Economic Policy (8.4 per cent), whilst Health, Nutrition and Population (6.5 per cent), Education (4.5 per cent), Water Supply and Sanitation (5.9 per cent) received less funding (World Bank 2000c). The types of investment and development projects the World Bank supports are either, large-scale 'sector projects' concerned with energy, transport, agriculture, forestry, rural development or smaller projects concentrating on education programmes, urban development, population measures, health and nutrient, water and sewerage treatment (George and Sabelli 1994; Abbasi 1999). The types of projects or loans funded until 2000 are outlined in the Table 3.1.

The effects of these projects and loans for the public health of developing nations present a mixed picture. Many countries have been instructed to change their methods of food production following the granting of Sectoral Loans from the World Bank. This has led to the increased use of pesticides, soil degradation, deforestation and resulted in major environmental and health problems for countries like Bangladesh that are likely to persist (Jubilee 1999a).

Table 3.1   World Bank loans and projects

- *Project Lending* Coal plants, oil development, fisheries and agricultural, dams, roads, education, health, clean water and sanitation.
- *Sector Lending* These loans govern the entire sector of the country's economy: energy, agriculture, transport and education.
- *Institutional Lending* In order to reorganise institutions, orienting policy towards free market and open access to trade markets.
- *Sectoral Adjustment Programmes (SAPs)* Intended to relieve debt crisis, convert domestic resources to production for export and promote trade.

Source: George S and Sabelli F (1994) *Faith and Credit. The World Bank's Secular Empire*. Penguin, London.

The International Monetary Fund (IMF)

The second Bretton Woods Institution created was the IMF with key roles 'to promote international monetary cooperation, to facilitate the expansion and balanced growth of international trade, to promote exchange stability and orderly exchange arrangements; to foster economic growth and high levels of employment; to provide temporary financial assistance to countries' (IMF 2001a: 1). In essence the IMF focuses on short-term macroeconomic problems (balance of payment problems) and has a key role in monitoring – in the form of surveillance or policing – the economic and financial state of member countries (IMF 2001a). The implications for public health are profound, as the role of the IMF is to promote fiscal stability and ensure that countries remain economically solvent, the result is that many of the policies imposed by the IMF have resulted in drastic reductions in health care expenditure, increased poverty and debt for many nations.

Initially the IMF only provided short-term loans to developed countries. However, following the international financial crisis in the 1970s the IMF expanded its role and started lending to developing countries and imposing structural reforms (Cavanagh *et al.* 1994; Wolf 1999a). Members joining the IMF originally valued their currency against the gold standard, which defined the value of a currency against a given amount of gold and the value of this against the US dollar. In 1971, the USA abandoned the gold standard and the fixed parity between the dollar and gold, and between the dollar and other currencies was broken (Branford and Kucinski 1990: 43). Currencies of different countries are now 'floated' and international financial markets determining their value. This can be a risky venture for countries that do not have a strong currency and has resulted in major devaluations in Mexico and East Asia during the 1990s and Argentina in 2001/2002. As the value of the currency falls so the money invested in health, education and environmental programmes declines, resulting in projects being insufficiently funded or closed and individuals having to pay directly for health care or education.

IMF members are now required to keep other nations informed about the value of their currency and to pursue economic policies that will promote national wealth and stability (IMF 1998). Currently, 183 nations are members of the IMF (IMF 2001a). A country joining the IMF makes a pledge to pay a capital subscription termed a 'quota' to the IMF, worked out on the basis of the country's wealth and economic performance. This forms the pool of money the IMF lends in the shape of credits or loans to member countries with balance of payment problems. Members pay 25 per cent of their quota in an international reserve (US dollars, pound sterling, yen) and the balance is comprised of the country's own currency or collateral, normally based on natural reserves such as oil, gas or coal which acts as a form of 'insurance' (IMF 1998). The quota paid by a nation determines the amount they can borrow from the IMF in the form of Special Drawing Rights (SDRs) and their voting power in IMF decisions.

Individually the United States has 17.16 per cent of voting rights, the United Kingdom, 4.97 per cent, Germany, 6.02 per cent, Japan, 6.16 per cent, whilst many of the African countries such as Burundi, Burkina Faso, Botswana, Mozambique, Niger and Mali have less than 0.05 per cent voting rights (IMF 2001b). The statistics for former Baltic and Eastern block countries portrays a similar picture; Poland, 0.64 per cent, Azerbaijan, 0.09 per cent, Romania, 0.49 per cent and Albania, 0.03 per cent (IMF 2001b). The consequence of this unequal distribution of voting power is that G7 countries, particularly the United States, dominate decision and policy making at the World Bank and IMF (Martin and Schuumann 1997). The lack of democratic governance and the limited power of developing nations to exert any influence means that the IMF can impose conditions (Wood 2001a). In order to receive the loan a range of 'conditions' are attached that include the implementation of a structural adjustment plan designed to reduce government public expenditure, tighten monetary policy and address structural weakness in the economy (IMF 1998).

The effects of fundamental economic and social change can be illustrated by Russia. Following the collapse of communism in the 1990s Russia received substantial loans from the IMF for structural reforms. The conditions attached included the abolition of state run public services and the introduction of market forces into the economy (Wolf 1994). The impact of these measures was substantial, the swift political and economic transformation resulted in fiscal decline, poverty and reduced health status (Hertzman and Siddiqi 2000: 809). Since 1990, average male life expectancy has fallen from 64 to 58 years, whilst GDP spent on health care in 1999 was only 4.2 per cent (Leon *et al.* 1997; World Bank 2000a).

A key role of the IMF is surveillance and policing of international economies to prevent instability in financial markets. The IMF undertakes a financial appraisal of a country's wealth and the factors that may affect long-term growth and stability. The IMF (1998: 8) contended that by undertaking surveillance or supervision 'strong consistent domestic policies will lead to stable exchange rates and a growing prosperous world economy'. However, in the light of a series of recurrent financial crisis since the 1980s the extent to which the IMF has achieved this aim has been questioned (George 1994; Chossudovsky 1997; Oxfam 1996).

International trade: World Trade Organisation (WTO)

Bretton Woods Institutions aimed to ensure economic growth and liberalise markets to prevent the protectionist trade problems of the 1930s recurring. The creation after the Second World War of the General Agreement on Tariffs and Trade (GATT) was intended to fulfil this aim and provide the mechanism for dealing with trade negotiations between member countries. In 1995, GATT was replaced by the WTO. Currently, the WTO is comprised of 137 countries, covering 90 per cent of world trade. Admission to the WTO is based on meeting a set of conditions, with most nations eager to access global markets and the benefits associated with membership. The role of the WTO (1999: 1) is to

- Administer trade agreements.
- Act as a forum for trade negotiations.
- Settle trade disputes.
- Review national trade policies.
- Assist developing countries in trade policy issues through technical assistance and training programmes.
- Cooperate with other international agencies.

The extent to which the WTO has fulfilled these aims is open to debate with some claiming that in practice the WTO works for the benefit of developed rather than developing nations (Oxfam 1996; Madeley 2000; Curtis 2001). This has profound public health implications because developing nations are unable to fund or sustain health care. The decision of pharmaceutical industries to exercise the WTO agreement on intellectual property illustrates this. Until recently, HIV/AIDS drugs in Africa were sold at prohibitively high prices that denied countries and individuals access to drugs they could not afford (Oxfam 2001a; Taylor 2001). Currently, there are 4.1 million adults in South Africa with HIV/AIDS, in Swaziland 25 per cent of adults are infected, whilst the number of children orphaned in Africa is estimated to be 12.1 million (O'Kane 2000).

Another major institution is the United Nations Conference on Trade and Development (UNCTAD) established in 1964 to help developing countries to reverse the decline in trade and to link trade to development. However, attempts by UNCTAD to ensure that trade is fairly regulated and to control the activities of Trans-National Corporations have been blocked by institutions such as the IMF, World Bank and WTO (Madeley 2000). Part of the problem is that promises of trade liberalisation that would allow developing countries to access western markets, particularly to sell textiles and agriculture, have not materialised (Beattie 2001b; Curtis 2001). Even if developing countries export other products they may still face insurmountable problems. UNCTAD (1998) has warned developing countries to be cautious before increasing their dependency on food exports since monopoly conditions are applied to many food substances and high tariffs discriminated against developing countries, meaning that access to lucrative western markets is restricted or denied.

International trade and trade disputes can affect a nation's economic expansion, particularly when reliant on a few products as its main source of income. The 1990s Banana Wars dispute, for example, between the United States and the European Union lasted for over ten years, escalating in 1999 when the former country threatened to impose trade sanctions on EU exports. The United States claimed its retaliatory action was in response to EU members continuing to import bananas from certain countries, which detrimentally affected American producers (Wolf 1999b). For many countries the banana dispute was catastrophic impacting on income generation, poverty, particularly where this remains the main export commodity and a key source of revenue. Currently, banana accounts for 80 per cent of the fruit consumed by high income countries, however, producers only receive 5 per cent of the profit, the remaining 95 per cent taken by retailers (*New Internationalist* 1999).

The debt problem for developing countries

G8 (G7 plus Russia) countries in 1998 promised to write off £70 billion of debt owed by the world's poorest countries (Tran and Denny 2000). The question of how so many developing nations become indebted, despite the existence of a range of international institutions reveals a number of contradictory policies were pursued. Evidence indicates that although some public health strategies did make a substantial impact, other measures were mismanaged.

One of the key factors that influenced public health initiatives was the debt crisis in developing nations and the strategies enforced by the IMF and World Bank to address this problem. Debt and debt relief have emerged as major factors causing poverty and ill-health and preventing health promotion strategies such as clean water, family planning and education from being implemented (Oxfam 1995; Caufield 1998; DFID 2000a). The 1997 *Human Development Report* (UNDP 1997) estimated that if indebted countries were relieved of their annual debt repayments, in Africa alone this would have saved the lives of 21 million children by 2000 and provided 90 million females with access to basic education. The issue of access to universal primary education was explored in an Oxfam report (2001b: 1) that found the debt burden of developing countries was still keeping children out of school. The irony being that universal primary education would cost $1.5 billion a year, yet countries will spend $1.8 billion servicing their debt. The evidence shows that illiteracy undermines efforts to improve health and nutrition; address the impact of HIV/AIDS and efforts to reduce infant and child mortality (Oxfam 2001b: 1).

The statistics indicate that from 1955 world debt grew from $9 billion to over $22 000 billion in 1998 (Madeley 2000). Servicing those debts – repaying the loan and the interest – cost developing countries over $200 billion a year, four times as much as they received in aid. In order to understand the impact of debt on public health it is important to briefly examine the history of debt in developing nations and the measures implemented.

During the early 1970s following a substantial rise in the price of oil, industrial nations experienced a recession. The effect on developing nations was devastating as the price of products such as coffee, rice, tea, cotton, which they relied on as the main source of income fell sharply (Oxfam 1995). This situation was compounded by the fact that countries had been encouraged to grow these crops by the World Bank, this resulted in a global over supply and depressed prices further. International banks started to lend more money to developing countries, who in some instances used the money to repay debts, whilst accumulating more debts to other lenders. Many bilateral and multilateral creditors, who were owed money adopted a policy of extending the period of repayment by 'rescheduling' the debt, whilst at the same time lending more money (Oxfam 1995). For many nations this resulted in a spiral of growing debt burden, as countries borrowed from a range of creditors to service the debt (George 1991; Cavanagh *et al.* 1994). A substantial amount of Mexico's debt in 1982 was owed to US banks and to avoid financial instability the American government intervened and underwrote the Mexican debt. Also, both the World Bank and the IMF were involved in providing loans to the same countries, replicating each other's work without a clear strategy or policy (George and Sabelli 1994; Oxfam 1995). To prevent a recurrence of the Mexican problem the World Bank and the IMF introduced a range of policies designed to address the issues but these had a substantial adverse effect on public health (George and Sabelli 1994; Oxfam 1995).

In summary the Structural Adjustment Programmes (SAPs) was designed to inject fiscal control, sponsor free-market policies, impose strict conditions and reschedule the debts. The SAPs cover the following area:

- Control of money supply.
- Reduce public sector borrowing and spending.
- Reduce government expenditure on social sectors.
- Introduce trade liberalisation.
- Reduce tariff rates and provide incentive for foreign investment.
- Abolish price controls.
- Privatisation public subsides.
- Withdraw subsides on food and other commodities.
- Wage freezes, deregulation of employment and job security.

Despite these policies world debt in the 1980s and early 1990s continued to rise from $0.5 trillion to $1.2 trillion, with those countries implementing structural adjustment being the most in debt (World Bank 1993). The effect of these measures for public health was substantial. The restructuring of jobs resulted in wide-scale unemployment, the abolition of price controls and the withdrawal of food and fuel subsidies has meant that many former Eastern European countries are experiencing increased poverty and ill-health (Leon *et al.* 1997). The problems confronting the developing world, whether due to poor environmental health or poverty, were also linked to the activities of the same agencies that purported to assist them. A central thrust of the SAPs was trade liberalisation, with the World Bank and IMF insisting that countries implement the policies outlined above if they wanted access to aid and debt relief (Madeley 2000). Evidence suggests that many of these loans were not a qualified success, rather than assisting developing countries, they have contributed to their economic plight and increased poverty (Ugalde and Jackson 1995; Creese 1997). The United Nations (UNDP 1999) estimated that if the money from debt repayment was redirected into health and education programmes the lives of seven million children could be saved a year.

In Africa every man, woman and child owes the developed world $357 and this debt remains the biggest obstacle to development and poverty reduction (Caufield 1998). The gap between developed and underdeveloped nations has grown, as countries are unable to invest in programmes designed to reduce poverty or stimulate development (Oxfam 1995). The implications for public health care provision are substantial as choices about health care are often determined by costs and access. Since 1980, developing countries have been exposed through lack of investment and infrastructure to diseases such as HIV/AIDS and have experienced a resurgence in TB, Yaws and yellow fever due to lack of treatment and access to vaccinations (Oxfam 2000; Drop the Debt 2001a,b).

Measures introduced to resolve the debt problem

The Jubilee 2000 coalition representing a range of NGOs was launched in 1996 to campaign for 'the cancellation of unpayable debts that will never be paid economically or will be paid only by exacting unacceptable costs in diverting resources from health, education and sanitation' (Jubilee 2000 1999b: 1). A combination of international pressures and the desire to mark the Year 2000 with a significant act spurred many bilateral creditors to call for a cancellation of all debt.

The IMF and World Bank were unable to resolve the debt crisis. Many of their policy initiatives had not achieved the intended aims and so they re-examined their roles in the 1990s changed policy direction (Abbasi 1999; Wood 2001a).

The World Bank Development Report (1993) *Health: Investing in Health* outlined a number of major problems with international health care systems that needed to be addressed if a reduction in health inequality was to be achieved. The key areas cited included the misallocation of funds, ineffective health interventions, the inefficient use of money, the inappropriate deployment of medical staff and inequity in access to basic health care (Abbasi 1999). Many of the problems identified were areas that had been funded by the World Bank and IMF development loans and SAPs to restructure. An internal review conducted by the World Bank revealed that only 17 per cent of completed projects in the health, nutrition and population sector contributed to the development of local institutions (Stott 1999: 823).

The failure to adopt appropriate measures can be illustrated by the approach taken to child health promotion in developing countries. Traditionally international agencies used an integrated case management approach to child health promotion, but for the strategy to make a significant and sustainable impact on child health, it must include social and environmental improvements (Ehiri and Prowse 1999). Available evidence (WHO 1995) shows that for most parts of the developing world, a significant proportion of the problems of ill-health and disease are closely linked to both environmental conditions and poverty. The problems confronting Tanzania, for example, are similar to those in many other developing countries – high incidence of infectious and parasitic diseases, low nutritional levels, and problems relating to pregnancy and child birth (Klouda 1987). There is acceptance (WHO 1995) that the primary cause of these problems is poverty exacerbated by, inadequate food intake, low educational levels, lack of safe drinking water and poor environmental conditions which adversely affect health. The brunt of the problem is borne by infants and children under the age of five, who although constitute about 18 per cent of the population, account for 63 per cent of all deaths (Klouda 1987).

In an attempt to address these issues the World Bank reorganised and in 1997 published *The Strategic Compact* which outlined a new policy direction based on poverty reduction and greater emphasis on partnership with developing countries. To counter criticisms that previous policies had been too broad and lacking in strategic direction four priority areas were identified to encourage development effectiveness (World Bank 1997: 1):

- Refuelling current business activities.
- Refocusing the development agenda.
- Development of the Banks knowledge base.
- Changing institutional priorities.

To support the strategic compact and ensure a clear focus on policy direction the Comprehensive Development Framework (CDF) was implemented (World Bank 1996). The CDF was intended to provide a more 'holistic approach to development' than had occurred previously and to replace the *ad hoc* Structural Adjustment Programme with the Poverty Reduction and Growth Facility (PRGF) and the Poverty Reduction Strategy Papers (PRSP). Both these measures were designed to achieve a balance between 'policy making and implementation' with stress placed on the interdependence of all elements of development – social, structural, human, governance, macroeconomic and financial' (World Bank 2000c: 1). For this approach to poverty reduction to be successful the World Bank argued that a transition was required from the development strategies, associated with sectoral loans and SAPs to a country-led strategy. The principles underpinning the CDF and which indicated the future direction for World Bank policies were (World Bank 2000e: 2):

- The country should own the development strategy and determine the goals, timing and sequencing of its development programmes.
- Governments need to build partnership with all other agencies.
- A long-term collective vision of needs and solutions.
- Structural and social concerns should be treated equally with macroeconomic and financial concerns.

The key policy implemented to address poverty was the Heavily Indebted Poor Countries (HIPC) debt initiative announced in 1996 by the World Bank and IMF. The HIPC is intended to relive the debt problems of the most heavily indebted nations (World Bank 2001c). The initiative was designed to be a comprehensive approach to debt relief that would make debt service burdens more manageable through a mixture of macroeconomic adjustments, debt relief and aid, however, few countries qualified and only after meeting strict criteria (Madeley 2000). The HIPC initiative reflected a growing recognition that previous debt reduction strategies had failed to make real progress and that an increased proportion of the GDP was used for debt servicing, rather than on health or education programmes.

In order to fund debt relief the G8 countries, various governments, the World Bank and IMF agreed to finance an HIPC Trust Fund (IMF 2000; Elliott and Brummer 1999). For a country to be eligible for HIPC assistance it must meet the following criteria (IMF 2001c: 2):

• Face an unsustainable debt burden, beyond available debt-relief mechanism.
• Establish a track record of reform and sound policies through IMF and World Bank supported programmes.

Forty-one nations were identified as requiring HIPC assistance, with the majority being African countries who owed a total of $200 billion (IMF 2000). Half this debt is owed to bilateral lenders mainly G7 countries, 37 per cent to multilateral creditors and 13 per cent to private creditors. Of these some 22 have been approved for debt-reduction packages, whilst some bilateral creditors have extended debt forgiveness and cancelled the debt (IMF 2001c).

Following criticism that the HIPC process was taking too long to relieve debt the system was changed. At the 1999 summit of the World Bank and IMF the 'enhanced HIPC initiative' was launched with the objective of 'providing broader, deeper, and faster debt relief, seeks a permanent solution to these countries' debt problems by combing substantial debt reduction with policy reforms to raise long-term growth and reduce poverty' (IMF 2000: 1).

Under the HIPC initiative all countries that borrow from the IMF, World Bank or access debt relief have to produce the PRSP.

The intention is that the PRSP are 'owned' by a country who are required to identify key areas for action, such as poverty reduction, and outline the macroeconomic, structural and social strategies required is achieve change (IMF 2000; IMF 2001d,e,f). The PRSP uses a framework based on poverty outcomes and the links between policies and outcomes are to address the following (World Bank 1999):

- A comprehensive understanding of poverty and its determinants.
- Choosing public action that will have the highest poverty impact.
- Outcome indicators which are set and monitored using participatory process.

The remit of the IMF is also changing, partly in response to the Meltzer Report (Summer 2000) which examined the roles of the IMF and World Bank. The report made a number of recommendations that included the need for a clearer delineation between the activities of the World Bank and the IMF, well targeted support for developing countries and for conditional debt relief to be given to HIPCs with a track record of reform. Although the IMF endorsed some of these proposals, a number of them were rejected. The IMF now intends to focus on poverty reduction, economic growth and ensure consistent policies are pursued. SAPs have been replaced with the PRGF which are the new concessional lending facility of the IMF, providing 10-year loans to low-income countries (Wood 2001a; IMF 2001g). The PRGF is intended to provide a clearer focus on the link between economic growth and poverty reduction. The following criteria are applied for PRGF loans (IMF 2000; IMF 2001g: 3) based on a country's per capita income – based on the IDA assessment of less than $885. Borrow up to 140 per cent of its IMF quota under a three-year arrangement. This loan is based on the condition of the country's balance of payments, the adjustment programme and the use of IMF credit. Loans under the PRGF carry an annual rate of interest at 0.5 per cent with repayment at the end of five years.

To counter criticisms that the PRGF are SAPs in another guise the IMF (2001f: 2) contends that they are fundamentally different. First, the PRGF makes poverty reduction a central goal, whereas this was an implicit aim with SAPs. Second, the relationship with the country's strategy is different, the argument advanced is PRSPs require a nation to develop their own plans for poverty reduction, in contrast SAPs were imposed by the IMF and World Bank. Third, the way the PRSP programme is formulated is different. The policy is based on joint preparation and assessment by the IMF and World Bank, previously this form of cooperation did not occur leading to duplication of both funding and programmes. Finally, the nature of conditionally is different with the IMF claiming to take a less intrusive role.

By March 2001, 77 low-income countries were eligible for PRGF assistance (IMF 2001g), but only four nations Burkina Faso, Mauritania, Tanzania and Uganda had reached the stage of having their PRSP reviewed by the IMF and World Bank (Tran and Denny 2000; Wood 2001b: 4).

The key question to ask is whether these initiatives have made a difference. Oxfam (1998) found that only a small number of countries had benefited from HIPC debt relief, whilst for the majority it was 'too little too late'. Countries such as Rwanda and Ethiopia emerging from civil conflict faced additional problems in receiving debt relief (IMF 2001d; Oxfam, 2000; Drop the Debt, 2001a; World Bank 2001d). The threats to food and water security, child health and health care through the failures of such schemes and their concomitant effects on public health in Africa are obvious and have been described earlier.

Poverty reduction in the twenty-first century

The issue of poverty reduction is a recurrent theme and a major challenge for public health in the twenty-first century (DFID 1997; DFID 2000a,b). A study examining world population and health suggested that the past 200 years have witnessed a revolution in global fertility, mortality and population growth rates, in which the demography and health of the human population has been transformed. However, vast geographical inequalities in health and income persist, and new threats such as HIV/AIDS, environmental degradation and population ageing have emerged (Raleigh 1999: 981). To address these issues, particularly global poverty and inequality the UN International Development Targets were established (Table 3.2).

UN targets provide a benchmark by which comparisons between nations can be made. Although progress has been made evidence

Table 3.2   UN international development targets

Economic Wellbeing
- A reduction by one-half in the proportion of people living in extreme poverty by 2015.

Social and human development
Universal primary education in all countries by 2015.

- Demonstrated a progress towards gender equality and the empowerment of women by eliminating gender disparity in primary and secondary education by 2005.
- A reduction by two-thirds in the mortality rates for infants and children under the age of 5 by 2015.
- A reduction by three-fourths in maternal mortality by 2015.
- A reduction by three-fourths in maternal mortality by 2015.
- Access through the primary health care systems to reproductive health services for all individuals of appropriate ages as soon as possible and no later than the year 2015.

Environmental sustainability and regeneration
- The implementations of national strategies for sustainable development in all countries by 2005, so as to ensure that current trends in the loss of environmental resources are effectively reversed at both global and national levels by 2015.

Source: DFID (2000a) *Better Health for Poor People Strategies for achieving the international development targets*. DFID, London.

indicates that many developing countries will fall short of the UN targets for reducing poverty and achieving a universal reduction by 2015 (World Bank 2001a). Kofi Annan, the Secretary General for the United Nations, warned of a loss of momentum in the international campaign for sustainable development and that many targets would not be achieved without real commitment from nations (Beattie 2002). A recent development to take forward this agenda is the New Partnership for Africa's Development (Nepad). The plan was agreed by the leaders of South Africa, Algeria, Nigeria and Senegal and is designed to forge a new partnership between Africa and developed nations and to cut in half the number of Africans living in extreme poverty by 2015 (Pank 2002). To achieve this goal, the plan envisages economic growth in Africa of more than 7 per cent per year for the next 15 years. This is double the Africa's average growth rate last year.

The International Fund for Agricultural Development (IFAD) calculated that only 10 million people a year manage to escape from extreme poverty, less than a third of the rate required to meet the United Nations targets. IFAD recommended the targets can be achieved by the better allocation and distribution of water to the rural poor, land reform, redressing the disadvantages of women and trade liberalisation for goods produced by the poor (Houlder 2001).

To achieve a sustained reduction in poverty and improvements in public health, the issue of globalisation has to be addressed (UNDP 1999). For globalisation to work DFID (2000b: 19) identified that two key areas need to be confronted:

- 'political will' because 'it is not inevitable that globalisation will work well for the poor – nor that it will work against them. This depends on the policies that governments and international agencies pursue'
- a more integrated approach to policy making.

For these strategies to succeed it is essential that the international agencies discussed in this chapter address this challenge.

Fundamental change to international institutions to tackle globalisation is now proposed (Viner 2000; Dodson 2001). Opposition to Trans-National Corporations is not new, but pressure groups representing very different views have collectively and successfully lobbied the IMF, WTO and the World Bank at their meetings in Seattle 1999; Washington 2000; Prague 2000 and Gothenberg 2001 (Madeley 2000; Dodson 2001; Tempest 2001). Elliot (2000: 1) reviewing the issue of globalisation contends that prior to Seattle it was assumed there was an 'inexorable logic to the process and that the market supremacist model would benefit rich and poor alike'. A thousand million people are still living in poverty and a tenth of them in the industrialised world (New Internationalist 1999). Currently, it is not easy to predict the outcome of these events or the effects on international agencies. However, the IMF cancelled a meeting in early 2001 due to concerns that protesters would disrupt proceedings.

The alternative question to pose is what would be the implications of not having institutions like the World Bank, IMF or WTO? The breakdown of the climate change meeting at the Hague marked an important point in global cooperation and stability (Gray 2000: 23). The argument advanced is that the whole structure of global governance – WTO, World Bank and IMF – is an American construction. Thus, without US involvement, reform of these institutions will not occur and the organisations undermined. The end result is that countries pursue their own agendas resulting in turbulent markets and the threat of protectionist policies re-emerges. In this scenario markets revert to the policies pursued in the 1930s, raising the possibility of greater financial instability and uncertainty in the world and so there is a need to ensure that institutions such as the World Bank and the IMF are maintained but changed to adapt to the new global environment.

Conclusion

The role and effects of international organisations on public health have been scrutinised. Evidence suggests that the attempts of many countries to break the cycle of poverty and debt have been undermined by institutions like the World Bank and the IMF. Many public health programmes have been compromised as nations and international agencies continue to promote policies that may not be appropriate for the health needs of a country (Ehiri and Prowse 1999). The change of policy direction by the IMF and World Bank in 2000 to concentrate on poverty reduction, coupled with debt-management strategies may achieve some real progress. However, there is a need to ensure that the strategies designed to alleviate poverty and provide public health are central policy measures.

At the Paris 2000 conference of the World Bank and the OECD the concept of a 'third way for the third world' was explored. This approach argued that economic development has to be more than growth in per capita income and should include 'pro-poor' growth that analyses macroeconomic factors in conjunction with life expectancy, access to primary education and health care (Islam 2000). The effects of adopting this strategy would be to measure the impact of structural changes on income and health and the well being of an individual and to recognise the key role that public health plays in addressing these issues.

References

Abbasi K (1999) The World Bank and World Health Changing sides *BMJ* **318**: 865–9.

Beattie A (2001a) Campaigners offer moral integrity for influence. *The Financial Times.* 17 July, 11.

Beattie A (2001b) The polite face of anti-globalisation. *The Financial Times.* 6 April, p 12.

Beattie A (2002) Annan warns on poverty targets. *The Financial Times.* 26 February, p 13.

Branford S and Kucinski B (1990) *The Debt Squads.* Zed Books, London.

Caufield C (1998). *Masters of Illusion The World Bank and the Poverty of Nations.* Pan Books, London.

Cavanagh J, Wyshan D and Arruda M (1994) *Beyond Bretton Woods Alternatives to the Global Economic Order.* Pluto Press, London.

Chossudovsky, M (1997) *The Globalisation of Poverty: Impacts of IMF and the World Bank Reforms.* Zed Books, London.

Cooper Weil DE, Alcibusan AP, Wilson JF, Reich MR and Bradley DJ (1990) *The Impact of Development Policies on Health: A Review of the Literature.* WHO, Geneva.

Creese A (1997) User fees *BMJ* **315**: 202–3.

Curtis M (2001). Global business too important to be left to business people. *The Guardian* 23 April, p 8.

Curwen P (1997) *Understanding the UK Economy.* Macmillan Press Limited, London.

Department for International Development (1997) *Eliminating World Poverty: A Challenge for the 21st Century.* DFID, London.

Department for International Development (2000a) *Better Health for Poor Peoples Strategies for Achieving the International Development Targets.* DIFD, London.

Department for International Development (2000b) *Globalisation and the Poor.* IFDD London.

Dodson S (2001) History of anti-capitalism protests. *The Guardian.* 1 May, p 4.

Drop the Debt (2001a) The poor who pay the price – the real impact of debt crisis (www.dropthedebt.org).

Drop the Debt (2001b) Debt relief problems require urgent solutions, say indebted country finance ministers meeting in London (www.dropthedebt.org).

Ehiri J and Prowse J (1999) Child health promotion in developing countries: the case for appropriate integration of environmental and social interventions? Review Article. *Health Policy and Planning* **14**(1): 1–10.

Elliott L and Brummer A (1999) Poorest nations to get $23 bn debt relief. *The Guardian.* 28 September, p 2.

Elliot L (2000) Global Megabucks plc faces setback. *The Guardian.* 14 December, p 27.

Field M (1989) *Success and Crisis in National Health Systems. A Comparative Approach.* Routledge, London.

George S (1991) *How the Other Half Dies. The Real Reason for World Hunger.* Penguin, Harmondsworth.

George S (1992) *The Debt Boomerang.* Pluto Press, London.

George S and Sabelli F (1994) *Faith and Credit: The World Bank's Secular Empire.* Penguin Books Ltd., Harmondsworth.

George V and Taylor-Gooby P (1996) *European Welfare Policy, Squaring the Circle.* MacMillan, London.

Gray J (2000) Wild globalisation. *The Guardian* 5 December, p 23.

Griffiths A and Wall S (1999) *Applied Economic An Introductory Course.* Harlow, Addison Wesley Longman Limited, London.

Hertzman C and Siddiqi A (2000) Health and rapid change in the late twentieth century. *Soc Sci Med* **51**(6): 809–19.

Houlder V (2001) Pledge to halve poverty by 2015 'doomed to failure'. *Financial Times.* 6 February, p 14.

International Monetary Fund (1998) *What is the International Monetary Fund?* IMF, Washington.

International Monetary Fund (2000) *The Logic of Debt Relief for the Poorest Countries.* IMF, Washington.

International Monetary Fund (2001a) *The IMF at a Glance: A Fact Sheet.* IMF, Washington.

International Monetary Fund (2001b) *IMF Members' Quotas and Voting Power and IMF Governors.* IMF, Washington.

International Monetary Fund (2001c) *Debt Relief under the HIPC Initiative A Factsheet. IMF, Washington.*

International Monetary Fund (2001d) *Debt Relief for Poor Countries (HIPC) what has been achieved? A Fact sheet.* IMF Washington.

International Monetary Fund (2001e) *Poverty Reduction Strategy Papers* (www.imf.org).

International Monetary Fund (2001f) *IMF Lending to Poor Countries – How does it differ from the ESAF?* IMF, Washington.

International Monetary Fund (2001g) *The IMFs Poverty Reduction and Growth Facility (PRGF). A Fact Sheet* IMF, Washington.

International Federation of the Red Cross and Red Crescent Societies (1996) *World Disasters Report,* Oxford, Open University Press, Milton Keynes.

Islam F (2000) Free trade gets a facelift. *The Observer.* 2 July.

Jubilee 2000 (1999a) Bring it all back home. The impact of debt crisis on all of us (www.jubilee2000uk.org/impact).

Jubilee 2000 (1999b) Who are we (www.jubilee2000uk.org).

Klouda A (1987) ' "Prevention" is more costly than "cure": health problems for Tanzania, 1971–81' in Morley D *et al.* (eds) *Practising Health for All.* Oxford Medical Publications, Oxford.

Leon DA, Chenet L, Shkolnikov, VM, Zakharov S, Shapiro J, Rakhmanova, G (1997) Huge variation in Russian mortality rates 1984–94: artifact, alcohol or what? *Lancet* **350**: 383–8.

Madeley J (2000) *Hungry for Trade. How the Poor for Free Trade.* Zed Books, London.

Martin H and Schumann H (1997) *The Global Trap.* Zed Books, London.

New Internationalist (1999) Bananas – The Facts. *New Internationalists* Issue **317**: 2.

O'Kane M (2000) AIDS: Welcome to the land of the dying. *The Guardian.* 8 July, p 7.

Oxfam (1995) *The Oxfam Poverty Report.* Oxfam, Oxford.

Oxfam (1996) *Oxfam White Paper on Aid.* Oxfam, Oxford.

Oxfam (1998) Making debt relief work: a test of political will Oxfam International. Position Paper. Oxfam, Oxford.

Oxfam (2000) The IMF and the Global Financial Architecture. Oxfam Policy Papers – Oxfam International Media Briefing 4/00. Oxfam, Oxford.

Oxfam (2001a). Drug industry price life saving medicines beyond the reach of the poor Press release 12.02.01. Oxfam, Oxford.

Oxfam (2001b) *G8: Failing the world's Children.* Oxfam, Oxford.

Pank P (2002) The G8 Summit. *The Guardian.* 25 June 2002.

Parkin M, Powell M and Kent M (2000) *Economics.* 4th edn. Addison Wesley, Harlow.

Peel Q (2001) How militants hijacked NGO party. *The Financial Times.* 13 July, p 9.

Pilling D (2001) Battle zones present last redoubt in war on Polio. *Financial Times.* 4 April p 13.

Raleigh V (1999) World population and health in transition. *BMJ* **319**: 981–4.

Stott R (1999) The World Bank Friend or Foe of the Poor. *BMJ* **318**: 822–3.

Summer, L (2000) Personal View: the troubling aspects of the IMF reform. *The Financial Times.* 22 March, p 20.

Taylor D (2001) Poor world health and rich world wealth. *BMJ* **322**: 629–30.

Tempest M (2001) Organised Chaos? *The Guardian.* 27 April, pp 1–4.

Turner M (2001) Where NGOs step into shoes government cannot fill. *The Financial Times.* 16 July, p 8.

Turner M (2002) Malawian hunger for resolution of crisis. *Financial Times.* 5 March p 7.

Tran M and Denny C (2000) Debt Relief. *The Guardian.* 21 July, p 20.

Ugalde A and Jackson J (1995) The World Bank & international health policy: a critical review. *Journal of International Development* **7**(3): 525–41.

United Nations Development Programme (1997) *Human Development Report.* UNDP, New York.

United Nations Development Programme (1999) *Human Development Report* UNDP, New York.

United Nations Conference on Trade and Development (1998) *Trade and Development* Report. UNCTD, Geneva.

Vaughan PJ *et al.* (1996) WHO and the effects of extra-budgetary funds: is the organisation donor driven? *Health Policy Plan* 11(3): 253–64.

Viner K (2000) 'Luddites' we should not ignore' *The Guardian.* 29 September, p 3.

Wall A (1996) *Health Systems in Liberal Democracies.* Routledge, London.

Wolf M (1994) Bretton twins at the awkward age. *Financial Times.* 7 October, p 19.

Wolf M (1999a) A new mandate for the IMF. *Financial Times.* 15 December, p 20.

Wolf M (1999b) 'Going Bananas'. *Financial Times.* 24 March, p 18.

Wood A (2001a) *Structural Adjustment for the IMF Options for Reforming the IMFs Governance Structure.* Bretton Woods Project (brettonwoodsproject. org).

Wood A (2001b) *Carrots and Sticks: A Quick Fix for IMF conditionally.* Bretton Woods Projects, Washington.

World Bank (1993) *The World Development Report on Health: Investing in Health.* World Bank, Washington DC.

World Bank (1997) *The Strategic Compact.* World Bank, Washington DC.

World Bank (1999) *Background and Overview of the CDF.* World Bank, Washington DC.

World Bank (2000a) *Entering the 21st Century World Development Report 1999/2000.* World Bank, Washington DC.

World Bank (2000b) *World Bank Group at a Glance.* World Bank, Washington DC.

World Bank (2000c) *Where does the World Bank get its money?* World Bank, Washington DC.

World Bank (2000d) *IRBD The World Bank's Role.* World Bank, Washington DC.

World Bank (2000e) *Comprehensive Development Framework Questions and Answers.* World Bank, Washington DC.

World Bank (2001a) *World Development Report Attacking Poverty.* World Bank, Washington DC.

World Bank (2001b) *What is the IDA?* World Bank, Washington DC.

World Bank (2001c) *The HIPC Initiative.* World Bank, Washington DC.

World Bank (2001d) *The Challenge of Maintaining Long Term External Debt Relief Sustainability.* World Bank and IMF, Washington DC.

WHO/UNICEF (1978) *Declaration of Alma Ata. Report on the International Conference on Primary Health Care, Alma Ata,* USSR. 6–12 September.

WHO (1995) *World Health Report: Bridging the Gaps.* Report of the Director-General of the World Health Organisation. WHO, Geneva.

World Health Organisation (2000) *Editorial.* WHO, Geneva.

World Trade Organisation (1999) *The WTO in Brief: Part 2 the Organisation.* Geneva. WTO (www.wto.org).

4

Doctors in Public Health – Who Needs 'em

John Middleton

Introduction

I am a Director of Public Health (DPH hereafter) in Sandwell in the West Midlands of England. I will describe my entry into the role, some of the historical baggage I carry, some of the principles I try to follow and the tools I use. I will also reflect on how practice has changed with the NHS reforms I have experienced. Changes are afoot as health authorities disappear and primary care trusts (PCTs hereafter) take on the mantle of public health (PH) guardians. The implications for the DPH role will be examined. Finally, I will discuss why the multidisciplinary world of PH needs its doctors.

My route to public health

I came into community medicine by accident. I had little idea that I might get a job dealing with these issues. My practice, and indeed much of the practice of the time was fired and inspired by the vision of Jerry Morris for the new community physician:

... the evolution of the community physician as epidemiologist, administrator of local medical services and community counsellor, professional man and public servant; his advent is in itself I believe a priority.... This is how the sanitary idea is evolving today. The barriers between clinical medicine and public health, between health officer and medical care administrator are crumbling. Public health needs clinical medicine– clinical medicine needs a community. In promoting the people's health, the community physician must be directly concerned with the mass problems of today and be able to draw on the community's resources to deal with these, not be limited to the categories of need or service that history happens to have deposited in his office. Incidentally it means a renaissance for public health.... Tomorrow's community physician will administer local medical services. But he can succeed only by building an effective intelligence system. Local epidemiology thus should be the frame for clinical practice and teamwork, provide tools for management and the improvement of services. (Morris 1969)

Communicable disease was regarded as of declining significance, the new public health problems were defined by Richard Titmuss, and Brian Abel-Smith and required epidemiologists to address the new epidemics of chronic degenerative disease, accidents, mental illness and disability using population medicine skills to address health and care service delivery problems. McKeown was also becoming influential in his description of the major influences on healthy public policy – better housing, nutrition and sanitation over and above the impact of the health services. (McKeown 1979) The Black report on inequalities in health was also simmering away with photocopies of photocopies passing like contraband from academics to bureaucrats and back; immensely influential but in a totally antagonistic political climate (DHSS 1980).

Tudor-Hart's description of the 'inverse care law' bridged inequality in health and inequality in health services; economic and educational disadvantages prevent access to good heath care.

The availability of good medical care tends to vary inversely with the need for the population served. This inverse care law operates more completely where medical care is most exposed to market forces, and less so where such exposure is reduced. The market distribution of medical care is a primitive and historically outdated social form, and any return to it would further exaggerate the maldistribution of medical resource .... A just and rational distribution of the resources of medical care should show parallel social and geographical differences, or at least a uniform distribution. The common experience was described by Titmuss in 1968: 'We have learnt from 15 years' experience of the Health Service that the higher income groups know how to make better use of the service; they tend to receive more specialist attention; occupy more of the beds in better equipped and staffed hospitals; receive more elective surgery have better maternal care, and are more likely to get psychiatric help and psychotherapy than low-income groups – particularly the unskilled. (Tudor-Hart 1971)

Local authorities rediscovered an interest in health, first deciding they needed their own health officers in places like Leeds and Oxford, to provide their own ammunition against service cuts, but gradually to start to engage in health protection and healthy public policy at the local level.

A brief history of public health in England since Victorian times juxtaposed with key reorganisations in the national health service is provided in Chapter 1 (Middleton 2002). Are we on a treadmill or an escalator? This history of slow PH improvement definitely places us on an escalator of improvement. But it is set alongside a treadmill of NHS reorganisations each one further limiting our ability to get on with the job of population health improvement. The NHS is such a political football that it is difficult to see how politicians will ever be able to resist tampering with structures. Managerial culture has tended to collude, believing change to be the norm, to be good and to be a goal in itself. Only latterly has anyone asked the question about the health impact of health service reorganisation (Smith *et al.* 2001).

DsPH need to understand – develop and use where appropriate – the following to protect their communities.

- European dimensions of local health problems (Lang and Whitehead 1997; ENHPA 2001).
- Wider global impacts of local actions and the challenges of globalisation (Navarro 1999; Middleton and Dimond 1998).
- Militarism (UNHO 1981; Renner 1990).
- Social inequality, (DHSS 1980; Whitehead 1987; Independent inquiry into inequalities in health 1999; ENHPA 2001; Middleton 2002a).
- Injustice and violence (Middleton 1998).
- Resources on effectiveness (Davies and Boruch 2001; NHS 2000a).

- Health and environmental impact assessment and ecology linked to sustainable development and the new economics (Scott-Samuel 1998; Ashton 1991; Stott 2000; Brundtland 1987; Middleton 1997; Boyle 1999).
- Quality of life and health status measures, and appreciate the limits of those we have.
- Power and the limitations of the new genetics. (Zimmern *et al.* 2001).
- Renewed knowledge of microbiology (Donaldson 2002).

Describing public health

The Acheson definition, first penned by the American PH physician, Winslow, in 1927, and subsequently adopted by the WHO in 1951 is one of a few I carry around and use. 'Public health is the science and art of the prevention of disease, the promotion of health and the prolongation of life through the organised efforts of society' (DoH 1988; Winslow 1951).

The sciences and arts are described in Chapter 1 and not all are regularly commanded by doctors in PH. Sir John Brotherston's utilitarian notion of PH as the 'organised application of resources to achieve the greatest health for the greatest number' can be useful (Draper 1991). A PH philosophy based on the Marxist conception 'from each according to ability, to each according to need' still merits further development. New economic notions of the limitlessness of resources, and that problems of shortage and deprivation are only caused by finite money, still need to come over the horizon (Boyle 1999). PH is about disease prevention, health promotion and the prolongation of life. PH embraces healthy public policy through primary health care, through hospital treatment through rehabilitation, social care and palliative care. Understanding about what works best is needed for conditions whether medically defined, like heart disease, or socially defined like loneliness, or politically defined like inequality. PH requires society's organised efforts not the organised efforts of doctors, not the organised efforts of nurses, or other health professionals, not even the organised efforts of health services, but, the organised efforts of society.

The DPH must carry around an understanding of notions of health, of causation of disease and distress and a knowledge of the means to prevent and treat these problems (Jenkinson and McGee 1998). I do, of course, use the WHO definition of health: 'a state of total physical, mental, social and spiritual wellbeing and not merely the absence of disease' (WHO 1978). The idea of social and spiritual health is important. In the context of the current rise in racism and xenophobia in this country and elsewhere, it is difficult to regard people suffering from epidemic hatred as being 'healthy'. Recently the WHO has reduced its aspirations for health: describing it as a resource for everyday life, involving the ability to satisfy needs, realise aspirations and cope with or change the individual's environment (WHO 1998). I like the Illich based notion, that health is 'self-developed coping ability'.

The task for public health

- to measure the level of health problems in the community
- to recommend the appropriate interventions to deal with those problems
- and to monitor the effectiveness of the interventions as they have been implemented.

In each of these areas there is an unfolding and almost limitless range and depth of knowledge and skills to be grasped and applied. Box 4.1 shows the ten competencies for PH, recently agreed by the Faculty of Public Health Medicine, the multidisciplinary PH group and the Royal Institute of Public Health and Hygiene (RIPHH). They are useful descriptions of what PH practice requires. Each competency brings a raft of individual activities from the complex – undertake needs assessment to the more straightforward – write a press release (Healthwork 2001). The Oxford handbook of PH practice is helpful (Pencheon *et al.* 2000) and Scally's progress in PH (Scally 1997). Draper's health through public policy is still an essential text on the role of public policy making in promoting or destroying health (Draper 1991).

Assessing priorities

The challenge for PH practitioners and the source of all potential conflicts comes in assessing priority – in dealing with a particular problem like heart disease or the relative merits of different health

Box 4.1   Faculty of Public Health Medicine, Multidisciplinary Public Health Working Group/the RIPHH developed through 'Healthwork' consultancy (Healthwork 2001)

---

10 key areas of PH working

1   Surveillance and assessment of the population's health and well-being (including managing, analysing and interpreting information, knowledge and statistics)
2   Promoting and protecting the population's health
3   Developing quality and risk management within an evaluative culture
4   Collaborative working for health and well-being
5   Developing health programmes and services and reducing inequalities
6   Policy and strategy development and implementation
7   Working with and for communities
8   Strategic leadership for health
9   Research and development
10   Ethically managing self, people and resources (including education and continuing professional development).

---

problems. On perinatal mortality for instance, what works can be anything from improving housing and nutrition and putting money into pregnant mothers' pockets to the way in which midwives record and act on intrauterine growth measurements. On coronary prevention, everything from inequalities in income to robust social support networks, to access and quality of coronary by-pass surgery. We could do less coronary by-pass surgery if we prescribed more statins, but we could prescribe less statins, if we prescribed more nicotine replacement, but we could prescribe less nicotine replacement if we prevented more smoking and we could prevent more smoking if we get the ad ban and keep boosting the price of smokes. But which should we invest more in, perinatal mortality or coronary prevention?

My practice in public health

The DPH must also carry around an attitude – you need to know what you do not know. So you must not be afraid to ask the simple, stupid or obvious question – you will often find when you ask it that the smart people do not know the answer. For instance, when someone quotes a percentage at you, 'of what?' is always a good next question. You need to have tools that will enable you to answer the question yourself. Having a working knowledge of critical appraisal of evidence should be everybody's business now. Having the where-withal to find out the answers when you do not know the answer is essential. You have to have the right retrieval methods, a good address book, organiser, internet or WAP phone and a suitably cultivated librarian. You have to build your contacts for local political reasons, for your own knowledge development and to maximise your own time management. The job is assessing health needs, advocating the right services and policies to meet those needs and monitoring to see that those services or policy interventions have achieved what the evidence says they should. This is analogous to clinical practice, it is also analogous to good managerial practice.

The community diagnosis – annual public health reports and surveys

The 300 000 people I serve are a very mixed multiethnic multicultural population, suffering some of the worst levels of social deprivation in the country. I regard myself as a doctor for 300 000 patients. I need to make a community diagnosis – through my annual PH reports (Morris 1969; Binysh *et al.* 1985, 1989; Middleton 1990; Middleton *et al.* 1995). I need to propose the remedies for the community ills, and I need to implement or recommend programmes to partners, that will improve local health. I will do what I can, and I will commission or influence what I cannot do personally.

The yearly PH annual report can be very powerful although to many DsPH it is a chore. Box 4.2 shows the main themes of 12 Sandwell PH annual reports. They become dull when they are only the 'bills of mortality' and do not propose specific action. They become ineffective when they are not tied in with planning cycles of health and local authorities. The report is independent and the editorial responsibility is of the DPH. Sandwell reports have covered such contentious issues as the possible effects of a nuclear attack on West Bromwich, conversion of military industries for socially useful purposes, and quoted Malcolm X. None were so outlandish that I would be alienated from my colleagues and the health authority. I have also used multidisciplinary, multi-agency teams to write many of the reports, the list of contributors is often more than 20. I can also be used as a mouthpiece for things that other individuals or organisations want to say, which I believe too, but they are not able to say publicly.

Box 4.2 PH annual reports for Sandwell 1989–2002
key themes

Life and death in Sandwell, 1989: overview of major influences on health, health service development recommendations and a proposed strategy for health for Sandwell by the year 2000.

Ten years to health, 1990: major economic themes; consumers of health? Vested health interests in tobacco, food, alcohol, shopping surveys. Community care act considerations.

Sandwell Health: the album, 1991: community produced annual report – voluntary organisation details, vox pops of attitudes and ideas of health, a primary school project set of letters to the chairman of the health authority telling him what to do about their health.

Sustainable Sandwell, 1992: major theme of sustainable development for health.

Sandwell under the knife, 1993: Review of five surgical specialities.

Sandwell under the scope, 1994: review of major medical conditions – diabetes – became a major focus for clinical guidelines and service development; asthma adopted by Sandwell health partnership as its priority for multi-agency action in 1995–96.

Safer Sandwell, 1995: major review of crime and PH – describing local epidemiology of crime. Regenerating Sandwell – a challenge or a lottery? 1996: review of potential to improve health.

A new deal for health in Sandwell? 1997: opportunistic report positioning Sandwell re HAZ bid.

Child friendly Sandwell? 1998: major review of child health issues including healthy public policy issues such as governance, child friendly town planning, and anti-bullying strategies.

All change for health? 1999: millennium special looking at changes in health since 1990, new initiatives such as changes in undergraduate medical training, patient power and community development, and WHO's Health 21 charter.

Hearts and minds, 2000: a review of the national service frameworks for coronary heart disease and mental health – their implications for Sandwell, interventions which affect both.

Neighbourhood health, 2001: A review of health surveys in Sandwell at local, town and Sandwell level, to inform neighbourhood management.

PH reports should serve policy and strategy and valuable educational and reference functions and be an archive. Many health visitors, local government officers, hospital consultants and students use these reports, particularly the PH common data set and demographic and economic data. I still refer on occasion to reports from my predecessors – to see how far we have or have not come. PH reports can also be used to pull together all the many health needs assessments, which a PH department will undertake in any year (Middleton 1995).

I have audited my PH report outcomes twice, generally favourably (Middleton 1995, 1999). However, 11 years after a recommendation to recruit a consultant in rehabilitation medicine there still isn't one. The 1999 PH report audited achievements against the healthy Sandwell targets we had set ten years previously. Good outcomes included clearance of derelict land, improvements in housing lacking a basic amenity, road accident deaths halved. Coronary heart disease deaths under 65 and lung cancer deaths in men were reduced by 30 per cent, breast cancer deaths by 18 per cent and infant deaths reduced, principally because of the 'Back to sleep' policy effect on sudden infant 'cot death'. All of these achievements greatly exceeded the healthy Sandwell targets we had set in 1990. On the down side, road accident casualties increased, lung cancer deaths in women increased and perinatal deaths remained at their unacceptably high level. I now regard road accident casualties in Sandwell as a major failure of my PH practice on all levels; it serves as a good example of how such an audit can be valuable:

• health needs assessment – we congratulated ourselves on the halving of road accident deaths and ignored the casualty increase
• policy intervention – we therefore failed to understand that cars were getting safer but driving standards have not improved and non-car users are more at risk
• partnership action – we have failed to form the right partnership to address road accidents – road safety has continued to be seen in Sandwell, as an activity within the purview of particular professional groups
• lesson – undertake the right health needs assessment reviewing all current information systems of police, local authority and health service and regional observatory, form a multidisciplinary group and devise a partnership strategy.

Policy development and advocacy

I have seen policy development and the practice of my department move forward on two main fronts – healthy public policy and health services policy. In the early days the healthy public policy section contained only health promotion practitioners and bits of other PH practitioners covering advice to local authorities, communicable disease control and programme areas for the care of vulnerable groups. With time our health promotion function diverged with a specialist community development for health team and specialist health promotion policy officers working in particular subject areas such as food, exercise, smoking and mental health. All of these programmes developed opportunistically over the 1990s. A community development function came about through the conversion of mainstream health promotion posts to locality officers working along the lines of Sandwell's social services and housing districts. The function developed using City challenge funding and single regeneration budgets so that by 1998 all six towns of Sandwell were supported by at least one community development specialist. The action for community health in Tipton team success persuaded the health authority to retain the expertise and moved the service on to concentrate on the deprived West Bromwich area (Middleton 1999).

The health promotion policy areas developed funding from regional and national initiatives – a drug and alcohol policy officer (Drug action team, DAT coordinator) out of the national drugs strategy, smoking policy out of regional tobacco control funds, other posts like mental health promotion had to be fought for out of mainstream development funds. A youth health strategy team was constructed from the caucus of peer sex education workers, originally funded from joint funding and HIV monies; once recognised and valued, a small group of youth workers then presented to the management team a compelling case for mainstreaming their work.

The suggestion that primary care trust DsPH will not be 'strategic' is startling – they will be loveable street corner familiar faces – known on the patch by health service professional and residents alike (Hunt 2001). Sandwell's experience of developing health promotion over the last ten years shows us that it becomes more strategic with time. Practitioners, partners and the public begin to understand the vested anti-health interests ranged against them and seek to influence policies at a higher level to lobby for national and international policy change, to act locally through partnership programmes and local agency policies. They shift their actions aimed at individuals, away from victim blaming and take-it-or-leave-it health promotion campaigns, and more towards collective community

responses, structured provision of information and peer educa-
tion/community animateurs/activists/'expert patients'/lay health
workers. They recognise structural barriers to health promotion
which require partnership approaches to bring about change. For
instance, exhortation to eat healthily in the food deserts of our
inner cities requires support to enable small retailers to survive
and second, stock fruit and vegetables. Sandwell's food policy work
shows how local health promotion can move from straightforward
provision – health education or 'razzmatazz' to a strategic policy
and partnership approach (Box 4.3). (Lang & Raynor 2002)

> **Box 4.3**   Sandwell's food policy development: how health
> promotion has grown up. 1988 – Sandwell's first food
> policy document launched based on COMA reports

- Schools poster competition produced some excellent materials some of which can still be seen in our meeting room but not much else.
- Healthy eating advice remained something which health promotion officers did as part of their duties throwing in bits of information when out at the health fairs and community shows. Dental officers and dieticians contributed.
- The first PH report for Sandwell recommended examining anti-health interests in the local food industry and tobacco retail. (Middleton *et al.* 1989; Middleton 1996) How many jobs would we lose if people stopped smoking? How many jobs might we gain through new healthy food product lines?

- The report 'In search of the low fat pork scratching' in 1990, gave clues about the scope for expansion of the local food industry (Maton *et al.* 1992).
- Seminars for local food manufacturers were staged with the sponsorship of the Black country development corporation.
- One recommendation, the development of food cooperatives, was successfully pursued through City challenge. We unsuccessfully pursued the idea of a food technology park and funding for a food industry development post through local economic agencies. These ideas are even now being rediscovered.

- Opportunistic funding produced a team of three community dieticians. We appointed a food policy officer, funded by the health service and based in the local authority environmental health department food section. Armed with extensive health-related knowledge and access to over 600 food outlets, this was a pivotal position for taking food policy forward.
- Four influential food policy documents were then developed covering commercial catering, hospital and nursing home, schools and

pregnancy and early years. Basis for the practical advice to workers in the field. Food policy officers have influenced, albeit insufficiently, two rounds of contract specifications for the school meals contracts. Food cooperative development began to show the potential for community care – services to the housebound, and sustainable development – interest in community agriculture with an aspiration to use local food to supply local food coops (Davis *et al.* 1999).

- Food coops and partners runners up in BBC Good Food Awards for community programmes for supplying many schools with healthy tuckshops. With HAZ we piloted the national five-a-day programme, developed healthy catering programmes and undertook food access studies.

- Food mapping produced greater knowledge of the extent of food deserts in Sandwell (Dowler *et al.* 2001). A dialogue has been opened with local traders – we intend to support them with retail cooperatives, supported schemes to buy in produce from nearby farmers in Shropshire and Staffordshire. Food cooperatives are barely scratching the surface of what is needed to promote healthier eating and much greater structural development and change is needed in all aspects of food retail.

- We have therefore supported local greengrocers and large supermarkets as well as food coops as suppliers for school fruit pilots. We have had one refrigerated store funded by the Regional Development agency, Advantage West Midlands and we are planning to develop further the urban–rural partnerships which will enable us to supply regional healthy fruit and vegetables at affordable prices. We are seeking further regional and European funding for these initiatives. We have contributed to the recent Food and farming reports (DEFRA 2002) and we have lobbied extensively for change in the Common Agricultural Policy which stockpiles fruit and vegetables and maintains prices out of reach of the food deserts of our inner cities (Lang and Whitehead 1997; DoH 1998; Middleton 1999, 2002a).

Forging partnerships in unlikely and difficult areas is rewarding. In 1990, closer working relationships with police had been a priority, now it is a mainstream activity. Our developing partnership with the Sandwell Traders Association in the context of food access is something we could not have envisaged in 1990. Partnership activity is essential core business for improving PH. Single agency interventions can be beneficial across a range of partner policy objectives and interventions by a single agency can help another to achieve its objectives.

- Improving the energy efficiency of housing will make homes more comfortable, reduce household fuel bills and put more money into the local economy, it will reduce CO_2 emission, it will reduce asthma and may reduce winter medical admissions and deaths.
- Traffic calming reduces road accidents, creates safer, livelier streets, helps neighbours look out for each other promoting children's play, community safety and community care and improves the environment (DOT 1996; Fletcher and McMichael 1997).
- The highscope early years education programme improves educational outcomes, reduces the need for social services and special education, creates healthier, wealthier, more successful adults and massively reduces crime (Schweinhart *et al.* 1993).

Alternatively, interventions introduced by one agency may have more benefit to other partners:

- Harm minimisation by drugs agencies has a powerful influence on crime (Marsch 1998).
- Random static road side breath-testing by the police will reduce road accident casualties (Dunbar *et al.* 1985; Rollings *et al.* 1987).
- Fluoridation by water supply companies reduces tooth decay (NHS centre for reviews and dissemination 2000b).

Partnership is necessary for general community regeneration (Russell and Killoran 2000). Efforts to regenerate areas solely by housing departments tend to create 'dormitories for the unemployed'. Efforts to eliminate drug and crime problems solely by demolishing unfit concrete jungles will simply disperse problems to other areas. Provision of new health service facilities in areas of high need without addressing economic and educational inequality of opportunity merely reinforce diswelfare and health inequality. All new service provisions without economic improvement is setting itself up to become a target for vandalism and decay. So partnership working is essential for PH improvement but has become a mantra. Partnership is a duty under the Health Act of 1999, so people believe they have to do it, even if it may not be clear why.

There are three structural preconditions, which assist partnership to be effective.

- Long-term relationships between officers at all levels of organisations statutory and otherwise, particularly at senior levels, enabling productive relationships to form and long-term strategies to be developed and seen through.
- Organisations must deliver their core business effectively. Partnership cannot take place while any partner is undergoing organisational change, battling with budget deficit or other service-related untoward incidents.
- Coterminosity is essential. Partners have to be dealing with the same client populations. On all these counts we have been going backwards, certainly in Sandwell.

Health services policy

Our department seeks to provide expert advice across relevant health services disciplines. Through the vehicle of a clinical policy advisory group we have since 1990, brought together clinical opinion from hospital and general practice nursing, dental, pharmaceutical, PH and epidemiology. We have overseen such developments as the integration of medical and geriatric care, development of clinical guidelines, served as the expert advisory panel for secondary care procedures into primary care, initiated strategy development on stroke services, pain services and intermediate care, psychotherapy services, management of self-poisoning, plastic surgery and wound care, to give just a few examples. 'Health services modernisation' and 'service redesign' have become popular phrases (DoH 2000b). Box 4.4 shows examples of some of the service redesign work we have been involved with over the last 12 years. A case study of the development of our approach to clinical guidelines is shown in Box 4.5.

The 1996 health and family services merger gave us opportunities formally to bring together the disciplines of GP medical advice, pharmaceutical and dental advice with other health service clinical policy specialists. Unfortunately, the artificial separation of healthy public policy from clinical policy making has begun to open up as PCTs are becoming established with each wanting their share of the scarce resource of medical, nursing and pharmaceutical advice.

Our PH management group contains consultants in PH, communicable disease, health promotion, community development,

Box 4.4   Health services 'modernisation' and 'redesign' in
Sandwell 1990–2002

Community mental health teams jointly managed by health and social services 1990. Merged ear, nose and throat services with hub and spoke model City and Sandwell hospitals, 1993. Joint commissioning manager for learning disabilities services manages pooled budgets from health and social services, 1995. Community drugs and alcohol services set up with planned withdrawal from regional low access/high intensity addiction unit, 1995. District hospital-based plastic surgery service set up, 1995. Nine months general waiting list target hit in 1994–95 (part of West midlands Regional initiative) Not sustained because of capacity – surgeons operating privately in spare time – lesson for present.

Sandwell General Hospital Geriatric and general medical services merger, 1996. Old long stay elderly care hospital closed; continuing care beds reprovision in private sector partnership, 1997. Winter capacity management whole systems approach successfully manages winter pressures especially 1997–98, 2000–present. (Poor in 1998–99 due to under provision in primary care.)

Discharge planning nurses expansion, CPN liaison service in accident and emergency and intermediate care developments, 1998–present. Expanded, modernised orthopaedic services turns around waiting times for elective surgery, 2000. Alcohol problem services in primary care, 1995–present. Hospital-based alcohol problem services, 2002. City–Sandwell hospital service, management merger, 2002. Reconfiguration of City and Sandwell obstetric and children's services, 2003. Reconfiguration of vascular surgery services, 2002–03.

pharmaceutical dental and nursing and general practice, clinical governance and information. This group addresses health circulars of the day, new PH problems locally and nationally and devises our own local responses. Community development colleagues have become more engaged in evidence-based practice whilst clinical governance staff have opened up to the power of user and community participation.

On being a DPH

Everyday is different, the range of material is vast and ever changing. The job beckons those of us who prefer 'jack of all trades, master of none', and to know 'vanishingly little about everything' rather than 'more and more about less and less'. PH certainly has

Box 4.5   Development of clinical guidelines in Sandwell

- PH staff member encouraged and supported to do a Masters degree in business studies.
- Project review of the pros and cons and methods of developing local clinical guidelines. This paper was considered by audit/clinical effectiveness groups who used locally agreed clinical guidelines as part of their forward planning for implementing clinical audit.
- Five priority areas for clinical guideline development emerged on clinical topics with common problems in primary care and in which considerable local expertise existed in primary and secondary care with willingness to move towards an evidence-based clinical guideline.
- Guidelines and implementation dates were back pain (1997) epilepsy (1999) peptic ulceration (1998) leg ulceration (1998) diabetes (1996). Each had auditable standards to which GPs were 'signed up'. In the case of back pain and leg ulcer management audits were carried out and measurable improvements in clinical standards were achieved.
- Further clinical guidelines followed – management of antidepressant care, prevention of falls and revisiting clinical guidelines on asthma and coronary heart disease management.
- During the implementation of primary care groups, independence of attitude by primary care professionals asserted itself, above all. As PCG clinical governance structures emerged, it became impossible to achieve consensus of approach or priority and difficult to get sign up to anything but the bare minimum requirement for national audit which in 1999, was expressed solely in the National service framework for coronary heart disease.
- Despite the existence of auditable standards and having the human resources to follow up outcomes of the care of patients, systematic follow up of these care programmes virtually disappeared. This provides a good example of how organisational and cultural change prevents progress on health improvement.
- Optimists suggest that primary care professionals have 'regrouped' and will exercise a wider degree of ownership for new guidelines that emerge in the developing PCTs. It has always been a problem getting professionals to agree common practice, even when there is plenty of evidence. So the question of ownership, which we addressed through the process of implementing clinical guidelines through audit was still not addressed sufficiently. A few more years have gone by and people will not have got the quality of care they should.

places for experts of many varieties. DsPH can call on and steer all the expertise, to manage professionals in such a way as to lead and adequately represent and interpret the expert information. The DPH then needs to be able to apply this knowledge generally, informing boards and the lay public on strategy; pulling together relevant expertise to manage acute PH problems as well. You have to lead and harness disparate professional and lay interests fairly and dispassionately in a way that each will accept, and through which each will entrust you to represent them.

Rehousing on medical grounds – 70 applications a week in Sandwell in the past – illustrates complex and 'tedious' problems with the offer of medical points to assist an individual or family up the housing priority ladder. This system was ineffective with people jockeying for position using medical conditions to assist their choice of accommodation, or people with severe health problems who would be unlikely to be moveable before they died. Sandwell planned out an algorithm that could be applied by housing officers in the routine course of their housing allocation – counting medical conditions as no more special reason for rehousing than fear for personal safety or closeness to sick relatives. We audited the outcome of the new system and found housing officers produced just as 'good' results as the PH doctors would have (Austin *et al.* 1993).

The DPH's job may be difficult and even dangerous. Difficult to place patients with anti-social personality disorders and challenging behaviour will turn up on the door with psychiatrists, GPs, neurologists denying or rejecting responsibility for them. A colleague was delivered a consignment of faecal material by an anti-fluoridation protester who had not paid his water bill in protest and been cut off from the water supply. Public meetings on unpopular hospital closures or service changes are always uncomfortable. I received a series of death threats from anti-abortionists after we introduced RU486, the medical abortion pill in 1991. The challenge of the job is in dealing with patients who are not ill, who do not see things your way, who do not have to do what you tell them. The interminable wrangling over structure and empires in each new reorganisation of the NHS is perhaps the worst aspect of the job.

Being a DPH is corporate, entrepreneurial and opportunistic and you need to maintain corporate responsibility. The idea of the independent PH practitioner giving independent advice wholly without cognisance or reference to other senior managers in health or local authorities is illusory. You have to be sufficiently influential with colleagues in those senior positions to be able to get them to act as agents to improve PH. Otherwise you will be isolated and ineffective. You have to be able to operate in such a way as to have 'earned independence' where your advice and actions are seen to be those in good faith, operating for the benefit of the population. This may mean argument and opposition to different interests at different times, and will not make you popular all the time, but your independence as an advocate for your community's health, has to be earned and respected. Sometimes this means that you will therefore have to make compromises and sometimes you will choose to do something that someone else wants you to do, something which serves their agenda more than yours. The problem which then arises is when serving their agenda becomes the only thing you are able to do. As a Lancet editorial suggested:

if the speciality is to flourish and if the directors are to do their job properly they will have to speak out on politically sensitive issues. The medical code declares that a doctor's first duty is to the patient (or in this case the community), not to the employer; doctors should be allowed to exercise professional judgement. Part of the reason that public health medicine has fared so poorly in the UK is that public health doctors have sometimes been seen as mere cogs in the machine. They tend to become visible only when they make unpopular decisions – they risk being execrated when they challenge some much cherished clinical practices or ambitions and they face dismissal if they challenge their authorities. Often they have not been given credit for very substantial achievements (eg. For the steady improvement in immunisation rates). Another reason is the eternal conflict between preventive and curative services. More than ever before, public health medicine needs a strong independent voice. In the arbitration between treatment and preventive strategies, public health physicians can expect to make enemies on all sides, not least from clinicians whose services are threatened. Moreover, they will be the perfect foil for politicians who are embarrassed by the lack of facilities for their constituents. (Lancet, anonymous editorial, 1991)

During the early 1990s UK health service managers looked to PH doctors to be the agents of rationing health care. The extra contractual referral – the means by which distant hospitals recovered income for treating your residents with rare diseases or requiring expensive care – became the time consuming yolk around PH doctors' necks. Much of the baggage that PH doctors carry – and much of the drive for non-medical directors of PH has come from the failure of NHS culture to let PH doctors do all of their job, and PH doctors' failure not to be so shackled. In Sandwell I have fortunately been able to develop both a healthy public policy arm of my work, and fulfil the health services expectations on rationing and clinical policy.

Part of the secret has been the appointment of outstanding practitioners. We have recruited and selected well. There are essential
managerial skills that PH practitioners of all description must have –
interpersonal and communications – verbal and written, recruitment and retention, staff development, team working, committee
and meetings management, record keeping. It is intensely professional knowledge-based requiring technical and lay-oriented skills
and expertise. It is necessary to understand why people believe
and act the way they do, you have to be able to put yourself in their
shoes and speak in jargon-free language where you can.

Public health: local government versus health service?

Place PH with local authorities and it resides where the majority of
the major influences on health can be addressed. The new duty of
well-being imposed on local government under the Local
Government Act 2000, suggests a stronger role for local government. Neighbourhood management and renewal is also a powerful force for PH improvement (Social exclusion unit 1998). Place
PH with health services and it is where the majority of health-
related professionals currently reside and where much of the
health intelligence can be gathered. The skills and competencies
of population health measurement tend to have grown up in the
illness counting industry, which has mainly been in the health service. The major influences on health may be outside the health
service – but we do not clamour for water engineers to be DsPH
now, because their bit of the health protection business is pretty
well taken care of. There is much to do to improve housing and
employment and reduce poverty. The actions required to do this
are in the hands of a range of agencies – national, regional, local,
statutory, voluntary and private. It is the DPH's job role to influence, to catalyse, to monitor and measure health improvement as
a result of specific interventions and partnership actions. We do
not argue for Citizens' Advice Bureau (CAB) managers to be DsPH
although they are potentially major contributors to health
improvement.

Successive governments have seen PH as an integral part of the
health service and now aim to give the health service a key role in
reducing inequalities and improve health. The same skills of

health needs assessment and judgement of effectiveness apply to ill-health caused by housing and housing remedies as they do to illness-treatment modalities. Governments see a need for local intelligence to implement health service-related health improvement and still to ration health care and limit use of ineffective treatments. As the health of the population has increased, and incremental improvement in life expectancy levels off, the relative contribution of the health services has become more important; it has been estimated to account for about 30 per cent of mortality reduction since 1975 (Bunker *et al.* 1994).

We cannot ignore the power of the health service to do harm. There are numerous examples of how PH approaches need to be applied to health services problems. Medical catastrophes require epidemiological surveillance, intervention programmes and monitoring; routine mortality and morbidity as a side effect of treatment or as a consequence of clinical error or omission is also a major cause of ill-health suggesting a need for PH systems of surveillance and control (DoH 2000b). Hospital infection is a more important PH problem than motor vehicles now. If the health service becomes a more important nidus for the spread of new variant Creutzfeldt Jakob Disease (CJD) than infected beef, there will be huge questions of quantification of risks and benefits, from health care. Antibiotic resistance threatens to render current highly technological health care practice obsolete at some point in the future (Donaldson 2002). In addition, the health service is a major employer, a major procurer of goods and services, a major land owner and health information provider. The health service can harness all these resources for health improvement or can function as a microcosm of unhealthy society in general – paying unskilled people badly, polluting indiscriminately and wasting resources. So, the PH discipline and direction has to be positioned somewhere between the health public policy and health promoting services and the treatment service.

Specialist PH is being encouraged in England to develop managed networks (Hunt 2001; DoH 2001). Currently these are unfunded, unsupported and merely expressions of goodwill between groups of PH practitioners to share expertise. There is no structure or accountability, no leadership or management and, unlike other clinical networks, they are not funded. They have been strongly advocated, with some justification where unitary local government covers four or five health service administration units (PCTs/groups). PCTs must have their own PH function but many of the skills are in short supply so must be shared. There are choices to be made and processes to be managed. The options are:

- the unmanaged PH network based on goodwill and existing relationships: the least administratively wasteful providing relationships remain good, personalities do not change and some-one-else's priorities do not get in the way;
- the managed PH network based perhaps on service agreements between departments for particular skills and policy areas: an administrative nightmare, requiring a committee of equals making bilateral and multilateral agreements; or
- some kind of formal structured agency arrangement. I favour a formal managed agency structure which positions specialist PH firmly in the middle ground between health services and local authorities. These can be funded jointly by health trusts and local authorities through Section 31 partnership agreements under the Health Act 1999. Wherever the local strategic partnership is – so should be a PH service. PH services agencies should be local strategic partnership (LSP) oriented and PH reports should be produced on LSP boundaries. Such an agency must not fall into the trap of becoming the only PH resource for an area – PH is everybody's business and the agency must be seen as a facilitator, a trainer and an information provider as well as a 'doer'.

Public health doctors: who needs them?

Edwin Chadwick recommended the appointment of district medical officers in 1842. It is perhaps ironic that Chadwick had such confidence in doctors at a time when the power of their science was so weak. Does PH need to be done by doctors? No. Indeed, most of it is not done by them. Does PH need doctors at all? Certainly yes. Does the DPH need to be a doctor? Not necessarily. All of the ten Healthwork competencies for PH practice can be encompassed in individuals who are not doctors. Most current medical directors of PH, myself included will confess under duress to not possessing all of these skills, certainly not in equal measure. And part of the skill is to be able to harness all of these competencies in the skill mix of your department. The DPH must be able to command the full span of knowledge of what works in addressing a particular health problem. In acquiring even this level of knowledge, an individual in a public policy field or a non-medical PH training is likely to have as many years in training or experience as a doctor.

Doctors bring a particular knowledge of the causation and experience of disease, a code of practice and professional commitment to doing the best they can on behalf of the patient (the community in this case). This emphasis on individual patient care may blind doctors to the responsibilities and challenges of population health. However, the medical PH training I have experienced has certainly ingrained these in me, and I see it in PH physician colleagues. Doctors I have known who have not been comfortable with a population health perspective and a public service ethic have generally returned to clinical practice.

Doctors in PH have been shackled by health service requirements, constraints and culture. Their bad press of the 1990s came from their complete diversion into the needs of health service rationing. But even now, if the health service remains the dominant culture in which PH must operate, there is no reason to believe that non-medical directors might not be so diverted. Indeed, they might be less able to resist.

Doctors are entrusted, licensed and empowered to take life and death decisions. In public administration we are all too complacent about the fact that we are making life and death choices. These are sanitised by the use of words 'priority setting' and even 'rationing'. As a doctor, I have been given permission to do what I do, through my training, through my professional regulation (much maligned) through the ethics of practice (however little formally taught) and the public entrusts me to do what I do. People accept what I say as a doctor when I am prescribing a population treatment as they might if I was in a consulting room prescribing for an individual patient. They believe I am making my recommendations because I have their benefit in mind. This is not absolute – it is not 'believe it because I am a doctor', because many people now expect to share therapeutic decision-making with their doctor, be advised, not instructed. This is not unconditional because people treat what their doctors say with healthy scepticism nowadays; and they are not ill, so I still have to use powers of persuasion. For most people it brings an air of confidence to decisions I have taken. The public may well accept other competent individuals and licence them to take life and death decisions but thus far I doubt if the public has really been asked. The public may require greater clarity of how an individual comes to gain such office.

In health service policy making and priority setting, where the dominant force is the doctors, and to a lesser extent nurses and other clinicians, the PH doctor does carry an advantage. The new PCTs need someone with skills and experience in clinical practice balanced with training in population and public policy approaches to health improvement. This could be a doctor, or a nurse, or another clinician. The PH physicians have been longest at it, and have the best developed training programmes. The case for PH doctors is persuasive. Politically of course, having a doctor on your side is immensely powerful in negotiations with doctors and other clinicians within health services. Someone up there thinks so too. The DsPH in the United Kingdom nations are all doctors, the chief medical officers. The DPH for the world, Gro Harlem Brundtland, is a doctor too although better known as a politician.

If the choice for DPH is between two absolutely equal candidates in every objective measure, and one is a doctor, I would choose the doctor. In practice, of course people are never exactly equal in every way. It is not an absolute: some powerful health service managers carry as many of the PH competencies and more individual clout than PH doctors. You would not wish to deny Edwin Chadwick or Florence Nightingale the chance to become DsPH. You would not wish to see Josef Mengele or Radovan Karadic given the opportunity. Public service ethic and the needs of the whole population is not always an easy concept for the doctor trained on the needs of the individual. The new DsPH will need to understand the ecology of health, new economics, sustainable development, and the global impacts of local actions; they will need to address the challenges of globalisation, of militarism, of social injustice and violence. In the particular circumstance, doctor or non-doctor will become less relevant. The judgement has to be made against the competencies required and the particular needs of the geography, the population and the tasks required. The appointed DPH must be the candidate with the most of the ten PH competencies, with the confidence, power and persuasion and with a public service ethic. Doctor or not. But there is certainly a role for doctors in PH – it is the role envisaged by Jerry Morris and still not yet fully realised. I will finish as I began.

> I have been personalising an individual doctor because in my own work I am very concerned with him, but of course this must be a team effort, involving several disciplines as well as physicians with varied competence. The traditional tasks of the medical officer of health as teacher, watchdog and trouble maker are being renewed, and he will also have new duties in the provision of services as an integral resource of health protection. One of his main tools will be knowledge, a contribution to social policy at every level. The community physician thus will be able to play his part in reducing suffering and in improving the quality of life. It is our good fortune to be able in this field to combine medicine and social science in public service. I appeal in particular to young physicians to join us. The opportunities have never been greater to give their best, use all they know and find fulfilment in service to the people and to their profession. (Morris 1969)

And again

> The best public health physicians will continue to generate action on local and wider issues. The task of public health physicians is to be well informed and to be brave enough to act on the information. If they are successful public health locally, nationally and globally will be greatly advanced. (Lancet 1991)

References

Ashton J (1991) Sanitarian becomes ecologist; the new environmental health. *BMJ* **302**: 189–90.

Austin D, Rao J and Middleton J (1993) Comparison of assessments made by a consultant in public health and housing staff on applications for rehousing on medical grounds. *J Public Health Med*, **15**: 346–51.

Binysh K, Chishty V, Middleton J and Pollock GT (1985) *The Health of Coventry*. Coventry Health Authority, Coventry.

Bowie C (1997) Estimating the burden of disease in an English region. *J Pub Health Med* **19**: 87–92.

Boyle D (1999) *Funny Money: In Search of Alternative Cash*. HarperCollins, London.

Brundtland G (ed.) (1987) *Our Common Future: The Report of the World Commission on Environment and Development*. Oxford University Press, Oxford.

Bunker JP, Frazier HS and Mosteller F (1994) Improving health: measuring effects of medical care. *Milbank Q,* **72**(2): 225–8.

Davies P and Boruch R (2001) The Campbell collaboration. *BMJ* **323**: 294–5.

Department of Environment, Food and Rural Affairs (2002) *Report of the Policy Commission on the Future of Farming and Food.* DEFRA, London (www.cabinet-office.gov.uk/farming/pdf/PC%20Report2.pdf).

DoH (1998) *Public health in England* (the Acheson report). HMSO, London.

DoH (1990) *Working for Patients,* white paper on the NHS. DOH, London.

DoH (1991) *The Health of the Nation,* white paper. DOH, London.

DoH (1998) *A First Class Service.* DOH, London.

DoH (1999) *Our Healthier Nation: Public Health,* white paper. DOH, London.

DoH (2000a) *An Organisation with a Memory: Report of an Expert Group on Learning from Adverse Events in the NHS.* The Stationery office, London.

DoH (2000b) *The NHS Plan.* DoH, London.

DoH (2001) *Shifting the Balance of Power.* Department of health, London.

DoH (2001) *Tackling Health Inequalities: Consultation on a Plan for Delivery.* DoH, London.

DoH and Social Security (1980) *Inequalities in Health* (the Black report). DoH and Social security, London.

DoH and Social Security (1976) *Prevention and Health: Everybody's Business.* DHSS, London.

Department of Transport (1996) *Traffic Calming Traffic and Vehicle noise.* Department of Transport, London.

Donaldson L (2002) *Getting Ahead of the Curve: A National Strategy for Infectious Diseases,* DoH, London.

Dowler E, Blair A, Rex D, Donkin A and Grundy C (2001) *Measuring Food Access in Sandwell.* University of Warwick and Sandwell health action zone.

Draper P (ed.) (1991) *Health Through Public Policy.* Green print/Merlin press, London.

Dunbar J, Ogston S, Ritchie A *et al.* Are problem drinkers dangerous drivers?: Tayside safe driving project. *BMJ* **290**: 827–30.

European Network of Health Promotion Agencies (2001) *The Role of Health Promotion in Tackling Inequalities in Health.* ENHPA and VIG, Brussels (www.vig.be/doc/kansarmen/Social_Inequalities.doc).

Fletcher T and MacMichael A (eds) (1997) *Health at the Crossroads.* Wiley, London.

Healthwork UK (2001) *Tripartite Standards in Public Health.* Report of the tripartite consultation on standards in public health. Healthwork UK for the Faculty of Public Health Medicine, Multidisciplinary public health group and the Royal institute of health and hygiene, London (www.Healthwork.co.uk/pdf/Public_health_consultation.pdf).

Hunt P (2001) *The Future of Public Health.* Speech to the Faculty of Public Health Medicine, London. 13 November (www.fphm.org.uk/Policy/Lord_Hunt_Speech.htm).

Independent Inquiry into Inequalities in Health (Acheson report) (1998) The stationery office, London.

Jenkinson C and McGee H (1998) *Health Status Measurement: A Brief but Critical Introduction.* Radcliffe Medical Press, Abingdon.

Lancet (anonymous editorial) (1991) What's new in public health? *Lancet* **337**: 1381.

Lang T and Whitehead M (1997) in Dahlgren Nordgren and Whitehead (eds) '*Health Impact Assessment of the EU Common Agricultural Policy*'. 2nd edn. Swedish National Institute of Public Health, Stockholm.

Lang T and Raynor G (eds) (2002) *Why Health is the Key to the Future of Food and Farming.* Health Development Agency and Thames Valley University, London.

Marsch, LA (1998) The efficacy of methadone maintenance interventions in reducing illicit opiate use, HIV risk behaviour and criminality: a meta-analysis. *Addiction* **93**: 515–32.

Maton K, Douglas J, Donovan D and Middleton J (1992) Food, health and work. *Local Economy* **7**: 64–73.

McKeown T (1979) *The Role of Medicine: Dream, Mirage or Nemesis.* Blackwell, Oxford.

Middleton J (1990) 'Life and Death in Sandwell', where public health and economic health meet. *J Local Govt Policy Making* **16**(4): 3–9.

Middleton J (1995) Audit of the Outcomes of five Sandwell Public Health Reports. Sandwell Health Authority, West Bromwich. Paper to the Health Authority.

Middleton J (1996) 'Converting Sandwell to a healthier economy' in Bruce N, Springett J (eds) *Research and Change in Urban Community Health.* Arrow publications and Liverpool university, Liverpool and London.

Middleton J (1997) Public health, security and sustainability. *Health and Hygiene* **18**: 149–54.

Middleton J (1998) Crime is a public health issue. *Med Conflict and Global Surv* **14**(1): 24–8.

Middleton J (ed.) (1999) *All Change for Health.* The 11th annual public health report of the director of public health for Sandwell. Sandwell health authority, West Bromwich.

Middleton J (2002a) Tackling health inequalities: what can health promotion do? European public health update. *J Euro Pub Health Alliance* **60**: 7–10.

Middleton J (2002b) Dr John's history of Public Health. *Public Health in Practice.* Palgrave, Basingstoke.

Middleton J and Dimond C (1998) Sandwell health puts on its SHOES. *Med Conflict and Global Surv* **14**: 331–36.

Middleton J, Srivastava NK, Donovan D, Rao JN and Douglas J (1989) *Life and Death in Sandwell.* First Annual Report of the Director of Public Health. Sandwell Health Authority, West Bromwich.

Middleton J, Pollock G, Binysh K and Chishty V (1995) 'How to do it: write – and use – the annual report of the director of public health' in

Reece D (ed.) *How to do it Volume 3*. 3rd edn. (fully revised). BMJ publications, London.

Morris JN (1969) Tomorrow's community physician. *Lancet* ii: 811–16.

Navarro V (1999) Health an equity in the world in the era globalisation. *Int J Health Services* **29**: 215–26.

NHS Centre for reviews and dissemination (2000a) *Evidence fro* Systematic Reviews of Research relevant to implementing the 'wider public h agenda. University of York, York (www.york.ac.uk/inst/crd/wph.htm

NHS Centre for reviews and dissemination (2000b) Systematic review o efficacy and safety of the fluoridation of drinking water. Centre reviews and dissemination, Tyork. Reprot 18 (www.york.ac.uk/inst/crd/report18.htm).

Pencheon P, Guest C, Melzer D and Muir Gray JA (2000) *Oxford Handbook of Public Health Practice*. Oxford University Press, Oxford.

Schweinhart LP, Barnes HV and Weikart DP (1993) *Significant Benefits: The High/Scope Perry Preschool Study through Age 27*. Monographs of the High/Scope Educational Research Foundation, 10. High/Scope Press, Ypsilanti (www.highscope.org/research/RESPER.HTM).

Renner M (1990) *Swords to plowshares*. Worldwatch Institute, Washington.

Robertson J (1985) *Future work*. Gower, Aldershot.

Rollings T, Middleton JD, Purser R *et al.* Coventry – A no drinking driving city by the year 2000? *BMJ* **295**: 71–2.

Scott-Samuel A, Birley MH, Ardern K (1998) *The Merseyside Guidelines for Health Impact Assessment*. Merseyside Health Impact Assessment Group and the Liverpool public health observatory, Liverpool.

Social Exclusion Unit (1998) *Bringing People Together: National Strategy for Neighbourhood Renewal*. PAT 4, HMSO, London.

Smith J, Walshe K and Hunter DJ (2001) The 'redisorganisation' of the NHS. *BMJ* **323**: 1262–3.

Stott R (2000) *The Ecology of Health*. Green books Schumacher briefing no. 3. Devon, Dartington.

Tudor-Hart J (1971) The inverse care law, *Lancet* i: 405–12.

United Nations Organisation (1981) *Report of an Expert Group on Development and Disarmament*. Thorsson report. United Nations, New York.

WHO (1978) *Strategy for health for all by the year 2000 (the Alma-Ata declaration)*. World health organisation, Geneva.

WHO (1998) *Health Promotion Glossary*. WHO, Geneva. WHO/HPR/HEP/98.

Whitehead M (1987) *The Health Divide*. London, Health Education Council.

Winslow CEA, (1951) *The Cost of Sickness and the Price of Health*. WHO, Geneva.

Zimmern R, Emery J, Richards T (2001) *Putting Genetics into Perspective*, *BMJ* **322**: 1005–6.

5

The Role of Nurses in Public Health

Yvonne Dalziel

Introduction

Research has indicated that poor health results primarily from poverty, the social circumstances of people's lives and the lack of control over the basics for survival, housing, access to food and warmth that material want creates (Townsend and Davidson 1982; Acheson 1998). This chapter acknowledges that the health service alone cannot address the huge public health agenda that is associated with these needs but suggests that nurses, especially community nurses but not excluding nurses in other sectors, could if they adopted a community development approach utilise a set of values for the development of a social model of public health – one that is about health and not illness.

Nurses have from their 'professional' inception often had a significant if implicit role in public health and fever nurses, school nurses, practice nurses, district nurses, community children's nurses as well as health visitors have worked in and with communities. In some regions of the United Kingdom still there are double or triple duty nurses who may function as health visitors, district nurses and midwives and who address a wide range of public health problems. Elsewhere in the United Kingdom and beyond there are WHO pilot schemes training family nurses who also look at public health matters. In the twentieth century there were some specific proposals to create 'public health nurses'.

The publication of *Nursing for Health* (2000) has paved the way for nurses in Scotland to begin to work differently, to move away from the medical model of health towards a more social and community development approach. It is often thought that community development is public health and that public health is health visiting. It is more correct to say that the methods, values and philosophy of community development offer nursing, and health visiting in particular, a way of addressing public health work. A community development approach to public health would put the community at the centre of primary care activity. It would support alliance working, working strategically and addressing public involvement and inequalities in health. The chapter shows how a community development approach can broaden the vision and capacity for social change by offering nurses the opportunity to begin to address the life circumstances that create poor health and create the services communities want. It suggests that there is no point in health professionals continuing to dictate what we think the public needs and wants. Rather nurses need to develop the conditions that support and help the public to have ownership of their own public health agenda. This relates to some of the approaches described in the research tools chapter.

However, the current structures in which nurses work will need to be addressed before community development can be used to its full potential; left untouched, public health nurses/health visiting, especially, will feel pulled in opposing directions. It will be more difficult for public health nurses to feel free enough to work with others while also attached to and part of the primary care team within a group attachment.

Nurses and public health

Public health is defined as that which improves the public's health. It therefore needs to have a population approach, to be strategic and to work in partnership with others whose activities also impact on the health of the public. Health workers often regard themselves as being the whole of public health rather than a slice of the whole. To be effective in addressing inequalities they need to join with other key partners in public health including housing, environment, police and education. The adoption of a community development approach could be far reaching in offering nurses a set of principles that will move the profession into a new era in its development. It will see nurses working with a health promoting and illness prevention model of health, working to achieve shared authority with their client groups. It will also demand different ways of measuring what nurses do. Outcomes may become less important than process and output measurements. Health visitors and others may be attached to a community working across practice boundaries to shift the energy and resources from medicine and illness to health. They will be accountable for their work and its outcomes not only to themselves and nurse management but also to the communities they serve.

Acheson's definition of public health cited in Chapter 4 has value. The science is the epidemiology and information gathering but the art is the approach to public health that nurses can use to engage the public in through involvement of the public in their own health agenda and in targeting their service to the most needy in society. It may be that contact with primary care services reinforces the feeling of powerlessness and low self-esteem experienced by marginal and disadvantaged groups. The adoption by nurses of a community development way of working within public health through primary care and other agencies that encouraged involvement and control by the community could shift the way individuals and groups perceive themselves and their ability to effect change. The process of gaining control of one's environment is then seen as being in itself health promoting. This way of working within public health could help primary care to begin to address the public health agenda in a way that encourages and facilitates a more involved response form the public. Nurses are in the community, they have skills and knowledge and because they work in very many different settings they have access to a substantial number of individuals and groups of people in communities. The Nursing for Health summary notes 'Community Development approaches that engage and build on the community's capacity for health will increasingly be a focus for nurses, midwives, and health visitors' community work...' (Nursing for Health 2000, 7).

A social model of public health

A social as opposed to medical model of public health would be underpinned by community development principles and have the following elements:

- *Doing 'with' and not 'for' ethos*: This is very hard for nurses trained to help and do things for people and often inadvertently creating dependency. When nurses begin to work with a community development approach it can be hard for them, because of the slow nature of the approach, and the fear of failure, to be unable to wait for the community to be ready to work jointly and instead to rush ahead and do things for them in the misguide notion of 'helping'. This happens when projects are starting and the community gets excluded from decisions like who and what to apply for in a funding application. Often this desire to help is couched in such terms as 'we need to know what we are doing first', 'we shouldn't raise expectations' or 'or it is too much to put on people'. Sometimes it is but more often it is not and the opportunities to create real involvement and individual confidence building are lost.
- *'Shared authority'*: Shared authority means the development of equal partnerships with communities where decision-making is shared. The Patchwork project described later (page 124) is a good example of how workers and users of the service can share all aspects of the planning and delivery of a service. Accountability is also shared. Shared authority demands different kinds of relationships between nurses and their users where personal and professional boundaries are constantly being negotiated.
- *Social capital*: The building of social capital in a community is very much related to the development of capacity through training for existing and new skills, supporting networks, creation of relevant services, involvement of the community in its activities and in decision-making. Nurses in the community using a community development approach will through using the notion of shared authority, empowerment and utilising the existing capacity of the community create social capital and improve public health.
- *Community defined health agenda*: Although a community development approach would support asking the community what it needs and wants for health the current obsession with doing needs assessments drains the resources, money and energy, needed to make the difference in community health. 'Analysis

paralysis' sets in. Often large-scale community assessment produces the same results: dog dirt, transport and crime. Important as these are they are often public accounts of health and do not begin to address what may be at the root of a community's difficulties; poverty, domestic violence, depression, alienation and lack of a meaningful purpose for life.

A community defined health agenda is more than a needs assessment it is an organic process that changes and develops and has at its core the energy, skills and interests of local people and their involvement as part of the solution and not just the problem.

Population/community approach

Public health is about populations and population groups rather than individuals. Acheson suggests that although public health affects individuals it needs the concerted efforts of society to bring about change. Thinking population rather than individuals may be difficult for some nurses trained as they are to deliver individual care but it is not possible to do public health with individuals. Public health nursing needs to be population focused. For example, contact with one woman suffering post-natal depression may lead the nurse to believe that the woman's depression is part of her personality or individual situation. However, collecting the stories or experiences of several women in the neighbourhood may begin to indicate larger social, economic or environmental factors that may need to be addressed before the problem is solved. Attachment to general practice makes it hard for nurses to have a population focus because practice populations rarely match geographical communities but instead chop population groups into individuals who happen to be attending a particular medical centre. One of the disappointments of Nursing for Health was the failure to address the conflict between nurses being group attached while expected to work with a public health population approach agenda.

Strategic and planned approach

Public health is about prevention and for public health to be successful in preventing disease and ill-health it needs to be planned and strategic. Community nurses attached to general practice may find it hard to work strategically when they are attached to a culture that supports practice concerns and practice populations and not geographical or communities of interest. To be strategic, nurses need to work together. For example, if child accidents are a problem in the area, one primary care team will be unable on their own to address the numbers of accidents that happen to children but will need to develop a strategic plan which may involve campaigning for safe play areas, speed bumps, provision of equipment like stair gates in homes and so on, and importantly the involvement of local families being part of addressing the problem. Public health nurses working at a strategic and planning level would therefore, in addition to working with mothers and parents groups and schools, need to influence local government departments, planners, transport ministry staff, the police, environmental health officers with a responsibility for home accidents, leisure departments, architects and builders. The work would also need to be informed by national and local statistics on children's accidents gleaned from hospital A&E departments, the Home Accidents Survey Statistics (HASS) and perhaps data from primary care settings too. How to identify, acquire and develop strategic and planning skills would additionally need to be included in public health nurse initial and continuing professional development training programmes.

Developing alliances

A key concept in the community development process is partnership and the building of alliances. Alliance is defined as partnership for action; a virtual organisation that is created by the interaction between partner agencies and sectors (Duffy 1996). The purpose of agencies working together and with local people is to develop common priorities and strategies on issues and policies that affect health. Partnerships for health work involve a wider spectrum than that usually associated with the health sector. For example, a health alliance would involve nurses working in partnership with agencies such as environmental health, housing, education, social work, voluntary organisations, health projects, work places and local industries. Funnell *et al.* (1995) identify five key features of alliance building (Figure 2).

Features of alliances building

These include the following type of activities, philosophy and tools to succeed.

- Commitment to the shared goals of the alliance.
- Community involvement in all alliance activities. Community representatives must have the necessary training and skills to participate equally.
- Communication where partners share relevant information and commit to simplicity, openness and honesty.
- Joint working with equal ownership and appropriate input from each partner.
- Accountability.
- Evaluation is built into alliance work and results used constructively (Funnell *et al.* 1995).

Successful alliance building also requires resources in terms of time, money, staff and commitments from all partners to achieve optimum results. Nurses are often disadvantaged in partnerships because they rarely are able to offer anything but their time and skills. Sometimes this is not enough and other agencies like community education are now beginning to demand that health meet their fair share of core funding for things like creches or hospitality rather than always expecting them to provide the resource.

Tackling inequalities in health: a nursing perspective

The Black Report (Townsend and Davidson 1982) indicated that it is the groups for whom the social movements had, potentially, the greatest impact, effectively those who are socially and economically disadvantaged, who are more likely to experience poorer health and have shorter lives than more affluent people. The community development approach to public health will build or develop the awareness of nurses about these groups. Such groups and others who feel socially excluded from mainstream society for instance the homeless and disabled, have important and often critical knowledge and experience about their own lives that when harnessed can strengthen and sustain their communities.

The dominance of the medical model in public health thinking and its focus on epidemiology and medicine has left a deficit in what nurses working in public health know about the poorest communities; what they need to promote health and to build the social capacity of their neighbourhoods and communities. Nurse involvement in public health work, through activities like community-based needs assessment, public involvement in primary care planning and delivery of services, would legitimate the community development approach and support the move to tackle the inequalities that exist in health and the access to services. The key tenets of a community development approach; collective action, self-determination, democracy and promotion of self-confidence are central to any policy to tackle inequalities in health and can cover the spectrum from the clinical model based on individual transactions to a social contract with entire communities (Ashton and Seymour 1988). To fit the new agenda of addressing social, as well as individual change in health, community nursing practice requires change in its approach to health as a concept and to the methods and the activities of its daily practice.

Although very closely connected and often confused as one concept, equity and equality are not the same thing. All people have the right to equal access to available health services for the maintenance and promotion of health but, to be fair, people do not all need to be treated in the same way. Instead, those who stand to benefit the most and whose needs are the greatest are given priority: this is 'equity'. In a culture of scarce resources, this may mean unequal distribution, even taking away from the most well off to give extra services to the most needy. All too often, what happens is the opposite; those most in need have the worst or fewest services. Inequalities in health care are not only about the provision of services but also how services are delivered. Addressing inequalities means challenging practices that discriminate against individuals on whatever basis: poverty, race, disability, language, sexuality or age in the provision of essentials for health. It also involves examining the provision, quality, uptake, accessibility and availability to those who have the greatest need. Public health nurses have an important role in addressing both inequalities and inequity in the communities in which they work. Some nurses, especially health visitors, find it hard to accept that the targeting of services and resources is necessary if the current inequities in health are to be challenged. Instead they defend their work with more affluent families arguing that these social groups also have problems. Of course that is undoubtedly true but better off people by and large already access a greater proportion of the time of health professionals. It may be that people who are perceived to be culturally and socially like them are easier to work with.

Promotion of health – prevention of illness

Labonte (1998) maintains that community development offers the best means by which health authorities can begin to tackle the determinants of health. The model he offers would provide public health nurses and other health professionals with a methodological and philosophical framework. It involves:

(a) the adoption of a model of positive health;
(b) an analytical model of health determinants;
(c) community development as a theory of social change;
(d) a model of community development practice;
(e) an accountability framework;
(f) development of methods appropriate to community development public health ethics.

Such an approach cannot succeed without the following elements.

Empowerment

Empowerment is 'the process by which people, organisations and communities gain mastery over their lives' (Rappaport 1984: 3). The empowerment process involves building individual and collective confidence and raising the esteem of individuals and communities through valuing their knowledge and experience and supporting them to be part of the decision-making process. Empowerment is also achieved through the attainment of 'participatory competence' (Kiefer 1983). Beigal (1984) views empowerment as both capacity and equity; capacity being use of power to solve problems and equity referring to getting one's fair share of resources. Empowerment skills include problem-solving, assertiveness and

confidence-building strategies. Nurses often talk about empowering their patients as if they had the ability to give people the power
they need. For instance, the giving of a leaflet is often described as
an empowering action probably because it imparts information. It
may be, but only if that person has reached the stage in the
empowerment process where that information can be used to
effect change and give them more control over their lives. The
information in the leaflet is not in itself empowering. It is more
effective to engage people in the empowering process by involving
them in decision-making processes, giving them a voice and valuing what they know and believe about matters that affect their
health.

Power and feelings of powerlessness can affect people's ability to
participate in a range of activities. Working on the power relationships within primary care may help participants to relate to the
difficulties experienced by the community in gaining access to
decision-making in primary care and to acknowledge that real participation in the democratic processes is quite difficult for many.
Community development is a way of working that aims to shift the
balance of power in communities and public health nurses may be
very well placed to support developments of these relationships
and processes but only if they are aware of how they feel about
power and authority.

Active involvement of individuals and communities in addressing health need

Participation is about supporting people who are affected by decisions and helping them to have some influence over their outcome. For nurses it is an important approach to the attainment of
health (Dalziel 1999). Perceptions of power affects participation.
Lukes (1974) suggests that there are different levels of power; the
visible manifestations of power, the unseen but tangible manifestations of power and internalised powerlessness. People on the margins of society experiencing this third level of powerlessness
become passive and dependent. Believing themselves unable to
influence events and decisions affecting their lives, they consciously
exclude themselves from opportunities to be part of the process of
decision-making. People who experience internal powerlessness

are often those who do not attend for clinic appointments, do not come to parentcraft classes or do not attend their children's school evenings. They do not believe their involvement can make a difference to their lives.

Participatory competence is a life-long achievement and should include three aspects:

(a) development of a more positive self-concept or sense of self-competence,

(b) construction of more critical or analytical understanding of surrounding social and political environment, and

(c) cultivation of individual and collective resources for social and political action (Keifer 1983). Nurses again may help over short and longer periods of time to foster and facilitate the development of such competencies in the communities in which they work as part of mainstream activity.

Consultation, which means a two-way exchange of opinions, is often used to determine health services and is an important tool

---

1. **Information Giving** – details of services, decision-making structures, helplines, media slots etc. This is a low level of involvement and is largely passive activity demanding little participation of the user.

2. **Gathering Information** – views on existing services, needs assessment, concerns about services, focus groups, community meetings. Again low level and fairly passive with little or no sharing of power with users.

3. **Consultation** – asking for comment on formulated plans or proposals. This has the potential to be power sharing but is often used when decisions have largely been made.

4. **Involvement in Policy Development and Decision-making** – getting users directly involved with management to develop training and quality standards for professional staff. This is the beginning of shared authority and can be empowering for users.

5. **Joint Working** – equal basis to develop projects, services, information packs, local forum, community health projects. This can be an empowering process for users and will increase confidence and self-esteem.

6. **Community or User Control** – involvement in planning and delivering services. This is shared authority and can be a very powerful tool for nurses in addressing inequalities in health.

Figure 5.1   Levels of participation or involvement

Source: Adapted from Taylor 1996.

for gauging public feelings on the development of services. Unfortunately it is often used when decisions have already been made and there is little likelihood of any change but the public is still asked to comment about a proposal. This is a poor substitute for real participation and being part of the planning process. Different levels of participation or involvement from information giving to user control have been mooted in a typography that is of use to public health nurses (Figure 5.1).

Nurses can support community involvement in any of these different levels. Involving people as part of the decision-making process is beneficial not only to the people living in communities but to the service providers. Giving users a voice in what they need avoids the mismatch of services and may be in the long run more economical for health services in terms of preventive and hospital interventions and treatments. This is discussed further in Chapter 1 and Chapter 11.

Primary care and public health nursing interfaces: a problematic past and partnership future?

The culture of fund-holding in primary care has left a legacy of isolation and actively not working with other professionals that may linger some time. Fund-holding did not support partnership and alliances with other practitioners, let alone other agencies or the community in which the practice was located. General practitioners (GPs) were encouraged to believe that they owned their nurses and often referred to community staff as 'my health visitor' or 'my district nurse'. Working from within general practice, with its small business focus and therefore some competition with other practices, nurses were often prevented from working with their colleagues in neighbouring areas because they might be giving benefit to patients from another practice. This is contrary to new thinking about health and public involvement and fragments community work. Nurses need to defend their right to work with geographical as opposed to practice populations and to be part of the move to shift resources away from practices to communities.

The benefits of community partnerships to nurses in relation to pooling information, knowledge, experience, skills and resources are too important to the promotion of health to be lost to medical politics. Joint working can be more efficient, effective and can widen and deepen the impact of health initiatives. In return nurses must be willing to share knowledge and power with each other, other agencies and, importantly, the community and to be involved in supporting community involvement. This will affect how they do community work. Our values, what we think and feel, will affect what we do.

The community development perspective may well challenge assumptions in primary care about its worldview. In a sense it directly conflicts with nursing and medical training where the focus is more likely to be on professionals who 'know best'. The first step might be to acknowledge that despite their training health professionals do not always know best about health and that individual people can be experts on themselves and their health.

Collective action

The author's and other experienced community development worker's experience suggests that the knowledge of what constitutes community development in primary care is very incomplete. Many health visitors maintain that they have been working in community development for years and learnt nothing new. They believe that running groups, giving input into a women's group or working with mother and toddler groups is community development. Small group work is an important method in community development and is to be encouraged but it is not the whole story. What is missing from primary care is the action part of community development. Concepts like partnership or equity are very palatable, empowerment is what many feel they are doing already but collective action is more threatening because it is about the transfer of power and control.

Collective action occurs when people act together to bring about the changes in their circumstances that they identify need to be changed. The women's health movement and radical groups of the 1960s and 1970s are examples of collective action. Today self-help groups formed around a variety of issues and pressure groups like disability coalitions or environmental groups use collective action to bring about change. When community development is working well the evidence of this is in visible collective action. Health visitors working with groups where they make the tea or put away the toys because that is what the participants want, must begin to question what they are doing to support empowerment and the development of social capital in their communities as a way of promoting health. With their colleagues they can adopt together a way of working that will create a level of participation that is more health promoting and will support social action in their neighbourhood to bring about change in community and individual confidence and self-esteem and begin to make a difference.

Refocusing health visitors as public health nurses

A community development approach is a useful way to move from exclusion to inclusion in the decision-making process for marginal groups and the principles of the approach could form an essential philosophy and praxis for groups of nurses. The approach is concerned with the notion of shared power between health professionals and lay people and the move from dependency to involvement. The concepts which underpin this approach are about equal access to resources, promoting democracy involvement in decision-making about health, taking action to bring about change, sharing power and working in partnership with communities.

Underlying each is the concept of shared authority. This means that each person takes equal responsibility for the decision-making and each is accountable for the outcomes. Although conceptually different each element of community development is related to and has an impact on the others. For example, when individuals are involved in equal partnerships and their knowledge affirmed, skills used and opinions heard, they feel more in control and are then more able to begin to form alliances with others to bring about the changes they desire.

Health visitors have been supporting a range of families, not just vulnerable families, for years and are increasingly being viewed, with other community nurses and school nurses, as an untapped resource for promoting wider community health. They are the ideal practitioners to take forward the new agendas in health such as 'Towards a Healthier Scotland' (Scottish Office 1999). They are in the community, have easy access to large numbers of families and individuals, develop the kind of relationships that engenders trust, and importantly, the principles of health visiting support them to work for policy change and to support collective action for health.

Meeting the public health agenda – challenges and dilemmas

The social or community development approach to public health offers a challenge to traditional ways and of working and may be met with resistance. *Thinking a Doing Differently* (Dalziel 2001), a report describing an initiative to integrate community development approaches to primary care and develop relevant training materials suggests that although there was evidence of change and a desire to work differently by many primary care workers the project found real resistance to new ways of working for a variety of reasons discussed next.

The focus of primary care work is geared towards meeting centrally imposed targets. The culture is therefore one of reacting to a policy driven agenda imposed from above. Taking time away from this kind of work schedule to work developmentally with a community to help *them* to identify their needs does not fit with ticking boxes and running a service that is determined by policy and practice needs. In *Thinking and Doing Differently* the participants discussed the problem of managing the conflict which can result from trying to work with two different sets of values and regarded this as one of the main difficulties preventing them from adopting a community development approach. There were also organisational and structural issues although there was some success in recruiting four teams to train it was not possible for staff to implement community development training into their day-to-day practice without the appropriate organisational structures. The community development approach takes time and needs to be properly supported to succeed. The need for organisational changes emerged during the developmental phase. The best way forward for the project and for this way of working required support in a variety of ways from senior levels within the Trust and the development of new support structures. In order to integrate new ways of working there needed to be:

- recognition within the NHS at all levels of management of the value of this kind of training and the community development way of working;
- consideration of practical support for the training including, how practice-based health professionals can be released to attend training;

- funding of posts for dedicated workers to provide on-going advice and support to implement the approach;
- further research to assess the health gains of such activities.

The project experience demonstrated that new structures and new posts to support training for primary care groups across practice areas in Local Health Care Cooperatives (LHCCs) needed to be developed if this approach was to be effective. Such posts would support closer working partnerships with communities and other agencies and would be an important way of meeting the new public health agenda. The project team was also being asked on a regular basis to give advice and support on community development issues to community nurses not involved in the training groups.

The role of GPs – a public health nurse perpsective

Some health visitors and GPs recognise that the community development approach with its emphasis on partnership working, participation of local people in primary care and shared accountability could support the public health agenda because it is a very good approach to tackling inequalities. The difficulty of getting practice teams together to train, due to lack of time and staff cover, presents a number of dilemmas. Should we work with those who are interested, regardless of their attachment to a specific primary care team? Is the advantage of working with people who are really interested in taking ideas forward offset by their potential lack of support without a practice team? Do we need GPs to be interested in community development training? Currently there is a question mark over the role of the GP's involvement in a social model of public health. Time, pressure of work and their own formal training seem to be key issues. In the report some practice health professionals said that they could expect little support from GPs, as they (GPs) are 'not very interested in things that take time away from practice activities'. That is not to say, however, that GPs would be opposed to community development public health projects or that they were unsympathetic. Their workloads are still such that they have to respond to busy schedules with a systematic way of working.

The difficulty some GPs experience in seeing the relevance of the community development approach was attributed to the fact that it is antithetical to their own training and to the bio-medical model of health. Some question the worth of involving GPs in the training and a number of GPs themselves, while supportive, could not see how they could 'get out into the community'. Rather, they felt that their role was to support and encourage initiatives. Community development is probably best understood through practical application. The Lothian project found that some participants saw a community development approach as an alternative way of working while others saw it as complementary. There is also a belief that a community development approach leads to an increased workload rather than alleviating pressure on overburdened health professionals. However, the training itself is an empowering process for professionals as well as the community. More emphasis could also be placed on promoting the value to the team of the personal development and the creative and problem-solving skills acquired through the training.

Impact on practice

Developing a different approach to community health and applying that approach to core activities is the main aim of the community development course. In Lothian there are now many initiatives arising from the training as practitioners begin to apply the approach to core work. These range from different ways of doing ante-natal education, working with parents in a drug project, changing baby clinics, developing local strategies for addressing CHD in an ethnic minority population, community-based alcohol strategy, men's health support, supporting asylum seekers and looking at befriending schemes for older people. Some initiatives develop well, others last for a while and then fold and some never take root.

A potentially exciting project called PEACH (Parent Education and Child Health) from one team showed positive signs of development. This initiative aimed to bring women with new babies together with women who were pregnant. The central theme was mutual support and peer education. There was interest from the local population but the idea never developed. There are many reasons why initiatives like this fail. To succeed with new ways of working, primary care workers need:

* support and time from a mentor who is familiar with the field
* appropriate resources (not always money)
* peer support to 'let go' and change practice
* organisational structures to support changes in practice
* a culture that accepts that failure is a legitimate way to learn.

Models of good practice

The Patchwork experience

This arose from the impact the training course and application of its principles can have on an area of core practice such as baby clinics. A group of health visitors in a disadvantaged area of Edinburgh were aware that the traditional service they offered to parents did not meet their complex needs resulting from economic and social disadvantage. After completing the *Community Development in Primary Care* training programme (described in *Thinking and Doing Differently*) they decided to work differently.

The health visitors followed the community development process and ran a series of focus groups to find out what the needs of the local parents were in relation to baby clinics. They then worked with this community to decide how they could achieve the necessary action for change together. A steering group composed of parents, health visitors, and representatives from community education and the local Community Health project was formed. The parents identified that to gain most from what the health visitors and local people could offer together they needed a place where:

* they could meet in comfort
* the older children could play
* they could meet other parents
* they could have tea and coffee.

The baby clinic was moved from the general practice building to the community centre. This shift from buildings that are medically orientated into community centres where the environment fosters social and community activities immediately created a more equal partnership and reduced the perceived authority of the health visitor. In this model of shared authority, child rearing was returned to the community where it rightly belonged. Health visiting activities then centre on working with the child-rearing constituency, lay workers and parents, to start the process of finding what needs they have. This is done not necessarily by formal needs assessment but by talking, forming support groups or organising discussions on child rearing or exchanges in which they are equal participants. Parents are part of the decision-making process and have an equal part in shaping what happens in Patchwork.

The Patchwork experience encourages new friendships amongst the women and reduces the isolation that can lead to post-natal depression. It acts as a source of information about what is happening in the community, encourages breast feeding support groups, and runs parenting groups around issues defined by the parents. These events promote good practice, help parents to learn about social relationships and support and help each other. The involvement of community education allows for educational programmes to be introduced and the parents now produce their own newsletter and are learning IT skills. The social action resulting from this new structure is currently concerned with developing local strategies to support ante-natal education and breast feeding that are culturally sensitive to that population and involve the expertise and knowledge of local people.

The uptake of traditional parentcraft classes run by health visitors and midwives is very poor. One of the Patchwork volunteers was interested in addressing this issue and, working with a local midwife, is finding out what women who live in this area want from ante-natal education and how they can be involved as peer educators. She has also started a breast feeding support network with some other women. This may make as much impact on local women as the breast feeding strategies currently devised by professionals within a cultural and social vacuum.

Valuing local expertise and knowledge around something as important as child rearing is part of building social capital. The acceptance of lay knowledge and experience alongside professional expertise strengthens partnerships with communities and will ultimately shift patterns of dependency away from health professionals and diminish community helplessness.

One of the lessons emerging from the project's negotiation and implementation experience was that in order to bring about organisational change there would need to be key interdependent changes within the Trust organisation and elsewhere to support different ways of working. These consisted of

- organisational authority for this approach to be implemented
- organisational structures to support the work
- change in culture
- relevant training to support the shift in practice
- support on the ground to shift the theory into practice.

Organisational structures to support the work

Changing the culture

Changing any culture is very difficult. One of the big changes for community nursing is that community development is by its nature developmental, whereas primary care is basically a reactive service based on professional knowledge and expertise. Nurses and doctors are trained to be expert and knowledgeable, a style of working which arguably encourages those on the receiving end to feel powerless, dependent and helpless. The community development training course encourages nurses to move away from doing *to* and *for* to doing *with* communities described earlier. Working more developmentally helps them see that local people, no matter how poor and disadvantaged, do have skills and knowledge. When harnessed, such skills can make a difference not only to their lives but also to the community in which they live. Health visitors largely welcome this change in culture. They want to reclaim their role in the prevention of illness and the promotion of public health. They are increasingly expressing a desire to be less associated with disease – supporting the work of doctors – and more involved in joint working with communities and other agencies with a community defined agenda.

New resources and new skills – shift in resources, training and education

It is important that nurses gain a body of knowledge and a range of skills that will allow them to be effective public health practitioners.

Some of the things they need to be able to do include:

- stimulate interest and response from communities
- elicit imaginative ideas and projects
- use the community development process
- involve the public in the planning and, where appropriate, the delivery of primary care services
- plan and run public meetings
- resource and support new work financially and in other ways
- work more developmentally
- develop partnership working
- manage the different relationships that will evolve with the community
- plan and run groups effectively and be involved in training local people.

Although it can be argued, and quite frequently is, that health visiting principles fit neatly with a community development approach, this way of working is very different from mainstream community nursing practice. Miller (1993) argues that in the process of change workers need to be given the tools to make some of the changes themselves. There is a dilemma for nurses in that in order that they can be involved in the process of helping others gain control they themselves need to move from immature dependency relationships with their employing organisation to relationships that encourage their personal authority.

One of the problems faced in changing ways of working is that when offered new methods they respond with 'we are doing this already!' Some of the confusion around community development arises from a lack of understanding about the differences between an activity that is community-based and one that is using community development principles. Community-based activities – mother and toddler or some women's groups – are often seen as examples of community development, but the absence of control by local people makes them community-based rather than community development initiatives. Moving from community-based programme to community development process is particularly important for community health nurses and health visitors, many of whom wished to challenge themselves by moving into an expanded and organisationally legitimate form of practice (Labonte 1998).

There is nothing wrong with community-based activities. They can be an important step towards local control and management, but if the notion of shared authority and collective action is missing then the activity does not embody community development principles and remains a community-based activity.

Nurses can contribute to the development of core public health activities. These would include:

- Building links and partnerships with communities and other agencies.
- Involving communities in identifying needs and shaping the response to that need.
- Setting up new structures, for example, food co-ops.
- Forming alliances with community groups for instance tenants groups.
- Developing social capital.
- Collecting meaningful data and spot trends.
- Getting involved with other agencies to address health need.
- Contributing to the strategic framework.
- Supporting inequality and anti-poverty initiatives.
- Encouraging community involvement.
- Working with community development approach.

The way forward

In Scotland, a new type of public health worker has been established in 2001, who may or may not be a nurse although most of those appointed have been nurses. These new staff are called public health practitioners and work in each LHCC in Scotland (Primary Care Groups (PCGs) in England). The role as described seems initially quite daunting, however, when various strands are applied to practice and to the everyday work in the neighbourhood they appear much more manageable largely because they are in reality interdependent.

The roles of the new public health practitioner

- *Providing leadership.* A key role for the public health practitioner is to provide leadership for the development of public health practice within the LHCC. For the reasons described earlier, changing culture and persuading staff out of 'comfort zones' to take on a largely new set of values and skills so as to become public health workers may create suspicion and be resisted. The health visiting service is a key area for change mentioned in Nursing for Health but other groups of nurses, midwives, practice nurses, community psychiatric nurses and district nurses also have a role to play in the new agenda. Change will be slow and needs to be accompanied by relevant training and support.

- *Address inequalities in LHCC population*: Although public health practitioners are LHCC-based in order to address inequalities the practice mentality must be avoided and instead a whole community approach adopted. The author is involved in a piece of work that brings together key workers to look at an 'inequality hotspot'. This is a small council estate located within a relatively affluent neighbourhood. Statistics suggest that 87 per cent of the housing estate is on some sort of benefit. Seventy-eight per cent of children attending the local school receive free school meals. This level of poverty suggests that there is likely to be very poor health. A suggestion supported by statistical evidence on rates of CHD, breast feeding and hospitalisation.

A group has been brought together comprising local activists, housing, midwives, schools, voluntary organisations, health visitors, community psychiatric nurses and police to start looking at what this neighbourhood has and what it needs to promote better health in its residents. A mainstream approach would suggest a lifestyle approach and that more information on smoking, alcohol and taking exercise would be appropriate but it is clear that this approach does not work where people are poor. Instead this group will look at some of the ways of addressing the life circumstances that create unhealthy lifestyles. One of the key ways is to reduce the poverty and so some of the ways may be to explore the expansion of the Credit Union, support people in debt, improve access to benefits, look at the role of businesses locally in creating opportunities for employment. The project will also begin the process of involving local people in addressing the needs they identify; gathering antenatal women and their partners and families together to look at provision of education and support, the development of a food co-op, organising some fun events to create a sense of community.

Working together we can develop the alliances needed to address the health needs and build the social capital needed to make the difference.

- *Develop health promoting alliances*: Public health demands a cooperative approach. No one agency can hope to do much to improve public health work on their own. The collecting together of other agencies like housing, education and the police and the process of beginning to help them see that they too have an important role in promoting public health and in the prevention of illness is a key activity of the public health practitioner's role. Health is only a small slice of the public health whole. Joining agencies together, coordinating pieces of work that would never have otherwise been done, connecting people with others doing something similar and making a difference is one of the most satisfying parts of the post. Contributing to policy development and evaluation and audit are also key aspects of the role.

These practitioners may prove to be some of the most innovative UK public health workers in public health nursing since the nineteenth century when their role has been carefully evaluated. The posts if properly supported, provided with adequate resources and given the appropriate authority will make a huge difference to the health of communities and the establishment of public health as a career for nurses and others.

References

Acheson (1998) The report of the Committee of Inquiry into the Future Development of the Public Health Function. Public Health in England. Cmnd 289. HMSO, London.

Ashton J and Seymour H (1988) *The New Public Health*. Open University Press, Milton Keynes.

Beigal DE (1984) 'Help seeking and receiving in urban ethnic neighbourhoods: strategies for empowerment' in Rappaport J, Swift C and Hess R (eds) *Studies in Empowerment: Steps Towards Understanding and Action*. Hawthorn Press, New York.

Dalziel Y (1999) *Community Development in Primary Care*. Lothian Health, Edinburgh.

Dalziel Y (2001) *Thinking and Doing Differently*. Lothian Primary Care Trust, Edinburgh.

Duffy S (1996) *Partnerships in Action*. Health Education Board Scotland, Edinburgh.

Funnel R, Oldfield, K Speller V (1995) *Towards Healthier Alliances*. London Health Education Authority, London.

Kiefer CH (1983–84) *Citizen Empowerment: A Developmental Perspective*. Prevention in Human Services, 3(23): 9–37.

Labonte R (1998) *A Community Development Approach to Health Promotion*. Health Education Board for Scotland, Edinburgh.

Labonte R (1998) *A Community Development Approach to Health Promotion*. Health Education Board for Scotland, Edinburgh.

Lukes S (1974) *Power: A Radical View*. Macmillan, London, Edinburgh.

Miller E (1993) *From Dependency to Authority: Studies in Organisation*. Free Association Books Ltd., London.

Nursing for Health (2000) Scottish Executive.

Rappaport J, Swift C and Hess R (eds) (1984) *Studies in Empowerment: Steps towards Understanding and Action*. Hawthorn Press, New York.

Scottish Office (1999) *Towards a Healthier Scotland*. HMSO, Edinburgh.

Taylor P (1996) *Public Health and Primary Care*. UKPHA, Birmingham.

Townsend P and Davidson N (1982) *Inequalities in Health*. Penguin Harmondsworth, London.

6

The Role of Primary Care in Public Health: A GP Perspective

Peter McCalister

Introduction

UK patients have most frequent access to the National Health Service (NHS) through primary care usually by making an appointment with their General Practitioner (GP hereafter): these are often called a 'family' or primary care physician elsewhere in the world. GPs and other members of the Primary Health Care Team (PCT) concentrate on improving the health of their patients but generally see each one as an individual. Until recently, few GPs would have been able to take a step back and look at the whole population of patients as a group. GPs and hospital clinicians are now being encouraged to look at patient groups for a variety of reasons that will be made clear in this chapter.

No professionals in primary care work in isolation. GPs, Health Visitors, District Nurses, Practice Nurses, Midwives and allied health professionals join forces to form the PCTs. I will focus on the role of various members of the PCT and explore the public health role of UK GPs. When examining the public health role of GPs, a number of problems become obvious. This chapter will set these problems in their historical context. Examples of the GPs' public health role will be given, and the problems will be described. Finally, some solutions will be suggested. The views are those of the author alone as a working GP.

Throughout this chapter I will refer to the NHS organisations which exist in Scotland. In the rest of the United Kingdom, the organisation, which I call the 'Health Board', would be referred to as 'Family Health Services Authority'. Similarly, the Scottish 'Local Health Care Cooperative' (LHCC) is roughly equivalent to the 'Primary Care Group' in the rest of the United Kingdom.

Organisation

History and 'the New Contract'

It is impossible to understand the present public health role of the GP without first understanding a little about how UK General Practice works. Nearly every GP in the United Kingdom is an 'independent contractor'. While each GP is employed by the NHS, he or she has a remarkable degree of freedom as to how the job can be performed with ramifications for public health practice.

As a GP experience, training, and motivation for the job are so variable, a variety of systems have been set up to make them a less heterogeneous group. Most young GPs now sit the MRCGP examination to become Members of the Royal College of General Practitioners shortly after their training is completed. However, this is not compulsory and most older GPs do not hold this qualification. Once in practice, GPs are instructed by their Contract of Employment to be available to patients for a certain number of hours per week to provide what is vaguely referred to as 'General Medical Services'. They have to perform certain compulsory health checks on their patients (such as a 'new patient check' and an 'over-75 check'). Apart from these requirements, GPs can spend their working life in whatever way they wish, concentrating on any aspect of medicine they see fit or, in some cases, just doing the work from day to day. Until recently there was no attempt made to re-educate GPs in any coordinated manner, with the result that services to populations are very variable, depending partly on the quality of your GP.

Coordination of GPs towards a common aim, such as secondary prevention of coronary heart disease for the population of a region, is largely achieved by financial rewards. There are clinical guidelines for GPs to follow, but use of guidelines has shown to be variable and generally disappointing (Baker 2001). Voluntary activity by GPs to improve the health of populations rather than individuals is generally achieved by spreading the word through the journals, which are read by GPs to a variable degree. Finally, the GP's immediate 'employer', remember that GPs are self-employed, is the Health Board with its Public Health Department and health promotion staff available to advise GPs.

In the days before the GP Contract of 1990, when GP recruitment was at an all-time high, many trainers and researchers focussed on the consultation with an individual patient. This led to a detailed analysis of the interaction between doctors and patients. New GP trainees were encouraged to explore the individual patient's physical, psychological and social problems. However, the government of the time was unhappy with this situation. Many GPs did not carry out all their tasks equally. Few had any knowledge of how many patients on their lists were suffering from common disorders such as asthma and diabetes. Many lacked accurate records of who was registered on their list. Computing was in its infancy although good software packages were being developed.

The 1990 Contract led to other initiatives which forced GPs to think of their patients in groups and not as individuals. This was unashamedly performed by splitting the GPs' pay into chunks and returning these chunks to the GP if he/she jumped through the right hoops. They were encouraged to perform certain activities, such as increasing the number of smears taken from a given target population and would then be financially rewarded. They were given targets such as 90 per cent of children to be vaccinated appropriately and only paid if the target was achieved or exceeded. GPs have since spent much time and energy jumping through the appropriate hoops showing how financially driven General Practice is. The amount of paperwork involved, the degree of Government 'control' over what GPs do, and perceived less time to see individual patients, are factors which have led to a catastrophic fall in applications for GP practices and training schemes.

From a public health viewpoint some of these changes were for the better. Audit has become compulsory and as a result GPs now know a lot more about their patients than they did before. If deficiencies in the care of asthmatics were discovered as part of an asthma audit, then these could be corrected, and the asthma clinic re-audited after an agreed period. As audits often showed that better patient management was going to be too time-consuming for GPs to manage, the numbers of practice nurses increased exponentially to cope with the new workload. Audit also became part of the training of GPs, and assessment in the MRCGP exam.

GPs were encouraged financially to maximise the number of childhood immunisations performed and the number of cervical smears taken. They were encouraged to take note of new patients on their lists and do opportunistic screening on these patients. Patients over 75 were to be offered an annual screening check, and all the rest of their patients were to be offered three-yearly health checks. Potentially the health of each GP's list would gradually improve and many previously under-diagnosed illnesses, such as essential hypertension, and diabetes, would be detected and treated. Some of these tasks, such as the three-yearly check, have since been removed from the GPs task list following pressure from the British Medical Association. The evidence behind others like the usefulness of the over-75 check has been questioned. GPs are now much more aware of what is happening in their practice population. However, each practice is still very different from its neighbour, even when practices share a town or the same premises. This leads to inequalities in the care that each population receives. If a practice wishes to become involved in setting up a Healthy Living Centre or invite Health Promotion staff to its practice meetings or involve itself in the local High School Health Education curriculum, then it may do so. However, many practices do none of the above and simply cope with the day-to-day workload. To deal with these differences, practices are now encouraged to work together in small groups (Localities) and in larger conglomerations (LHCCs and Primary Care Groups or Primary Care Trusts in England). When groups of professionals meet in larger numbers, there are many occasions where agreement between them becomes more difficult.

The 'independent contractor' status of GPs has been questioned and may vanish despite GP resistance. The development of new

GPs who provide 'Personal Medical Services' to a population, or works for a salary may be beneficial to public health. GPs would become more accountable to Government, and inequalities in GP behaviour would begin to be reduced. Some of the innovative services which the independent contractor status allows could also be stifled and UK General Practice may be so vibrant because it is independent. Care needs to be taken to ensure the restrictive New Contract is not replaced by another restrictive list of tasks to be performed as part of Personal Medical Services contracts.

Audit has become compulsory for all GPs and many find that it is not as terrible as it sounds but there is a financial price to pay which needs to be set against audit benefits (Lough 2000). As each practice, Locality and LHCC, become better informed about its population of patients, changes can be made to improve services appropriately. On a regional or national scale, projects such as the Continuous Morbidity Recording in Scotland should lead to a better understanding of the true prevalence of acute and chronic illnesses. The United Kingdom is fortunate in having a relatively robust and developed primary care system, which has been shown to make a major contribution to reductions in mortality in populations. In contrast, countries with poor primary care have, on average, poorer health outcomes, although there are important caveats depending on other characteristics of the countries. If health indicators such as neonatal mortality, infant mortality, mortality rates and suicide rates, are compared between countries, those countries with well-developed primary care systems like the United Kingdom, the Netherlands and Denmark fare better than those without such as Belgium, France and the United States. The former also have lower overall health care costs. Within countries, areas with higher primary care physician availability have healthier populations. More primary care availability also reduces the adverse effects of social inequality (Starfield 2001).

The US health care system is lavishly funded and those with adequate insurance usually receive excellent attention. But the system is fragmented and inequitable with little emphasis on population care. The development of LHCCs and Primary Care Groups in the United Kingdom, however, while offering the opportunity of better integration with public health and social services, may threaten the British GPs' role as independent advocates by giving them a rationing role. Managed care has forced a similar role on doctors in the United States, with consequent public displeasure and professional disillusion. UK GPs need to steer a careful course if they are to avoid a similar fate (Koperski 2000). In summary, it seems there is public health evidence for fostering a strong primary care system.

Health Promotion – the effect of financial carrots on sticks

The control of GPs by financial incentives can lead to chaos, for instance, through the encouragement of 'Health Promotion' during the 1990s. In 1990, the Contract rewarded GPs with a fee for every patient seen in a Health Promotion Clinic that practices could set up as they saw fit. GPs therefore set up Well Woman Clinics, Well Man Clinics, Asthma Clinics, Diabetic Clinics and Menopause Clinics. Many of these were staffed by Practice Nurses who performed certain checks and gave out advice leaflets if required. The useful clinics survived – such as asthma clinics, diabetic clinics and well woman clinics – as they fulfilled a need in the population and helped organise shared care with hospital colleagues. Some non-specific condition clinics set up simply to make money failed. For example, if GPs could gather together six anxious people, and look at their anxiety in some sort of structured way, this became a Stress Management Clinic, and GPs claimed a fee. Government grew suspicious about the massive rise in clinics and the system changed. All patients aged 20–65 were 'offered health promotion' by having their height, weight and blood pressure measured, and alcohol/smoking habits recorded. Advice was to be given where appropriate on such things as diet.

This new system was pursued with vigour by GPs to attract the fees available. Practice computer systems were set up to monitor how many of the prescribed population had been measured each year, notes were flagged, and a weighty annual report sent to the Health Board. Data about practice populations were gathered though evidence on its public health usefulness was meagre. Eventually the new system also became unwieldy, with annual reports too difficult for Health Boards to assess. The plan was once again changed. Practices did not have to produce Annual Reports but a 'Practice Development Plan' with little health promotion emphasis. Yet, by producing this Plan each GP would receive Health Promotion fees, which s/he had striven for under the previous two systems.

Did this improve public health? Only the 'worried well' attended the Health Promotion clinics and subsequent health checks. Those really needing advice on their diet, smoking or alcohol consumption stayed away. The ill-thought-out initiatives created an atmosphere of dislike in GP circles for the term 'Health Promotion'. Most GPs felt they were providing this on an individual patient basis and disliked 'number crunching' and producing reports. Health Promotion is still a low priority for many GPs. A WHO questionnaire survey of over 2300 GPs in 16 countries identified four main barriers to preventive medicine: unsupportive government health policies; insufficient training; lack of payment; and time constraints (WHO 1998). Financial incentives alone are clearly not enough to improve public health.

Information

The Practice Development Plan may still provide a happy ending from a public health viewpoint. Practices are now encouraged to collect data which include numbers of patients with coronary heart disease, asthma, certain cancers and other prevalent illnesses. This encourages these practices to look at the size of the problems in their area, and also provides the first nationwide census of the prevalence of these conditions in primary care. Practices can then identify those diseases that need attention, particularly from a public health viewpoint, and help them plan workload. The information will find its way to public health departments who will have a more accurate database for the health of the population.

The value of epidemiological information is dependent on the accuracy of data collected. Primary care clinical information is collected in a myriad of different ways and put on various paper-based or computer systems. Seldom are these systems united in locality, regional or national audits. Thus, if we ask a simple question such as 'what is the incidence of chronic bronchitis in the community?' the answer is unknown. GPs who wish to plan their drug budgets, nursing services, and assess workload cannot then do so easily. Increased computer usage in GP practice has allowed large amounts of clinical information to be collected. If GP practices so wish, they can provide detailed information on the prevalence of disease, and the amount of workload each illness creates in primary care. This has obvious repercussions for planning of services. These projects are not yet compulsory. There are still errors in recording of information but the use of Information Technology in primary care will certainly improve the accuracy of public health data.

Guidelines

Guidelines for the diagnosis, investigation and management of many illnesses have been produced by many agencies in the last decade. These are designed to reduce inequalities in health and guide GPs who cannot keep abreast of all research findings by offering critiques and summaries of relevant evidence in a readable form. The number of guidelines has increased to such an extent that it is difficult to read all of them and many give conflicting advice on the same topic. GPs may also lose the ability to read and analyse the evidence themselves and a 'dumbing-down' effect will occur.

Guidelines are, however, not directives and the independent contractor status of GPs allows them to exercise clinical judgement which may at times contradict guidelines. Organisations such as NICE (the National Institute for Clinical Excellence) in England and Wales are attempting to disseminate a balanced view of the evidence on a number of health topics for GP and other clinician action. If this succeeds, differences between GP practices should end as should the 'post code lottery' whereby different patients receive different care, depending on where they live. NICE therefore has an important public health role in controlling GP action but GPs may not accept NICE guidelines where the average patient in a GP surgery does not fit into a guideline developed by a committee consisting mainly of secondary care clinicians.

Hospital offloading

This refers to the care of patients in the community who were previously cared for by hospital staff. This happens in almost every field of communication between primary and secondary care, and has been a source of complaint that the resources to manage the patient do not 'follow the patient'. GPs have little or no say in the provision of services in secondary care in Scotland. Elsewhere in the United Kingdom they do have some power in the commissioning of care but the whole of the United Kingdom has suffered from relentless hospital closures since the 1980s.

If the GP looks at his or her public health role in hospital offloading, several points become important. First, the closure of large Psychiatric Hospitals has led to the care in the community system, where GPs form part of the team to care for larger numbers of mentally ill individuals. This includes those with learning disabilities and a variety of psychiatric patients, some who may be a danger to themselves and others in the community. Not all GPs are trained in psychiatry and, if they have a role to play in supervising these vulnerable individuals, they may not be able to fulfil that role adequately.

Where community care has succeeded, these individuals do not consult their GP regularly and few GPs have a rolling programme of reviewing them regularly. An alarming number has dropped out of the system and become homeless vagrants. Estimates vary but mental illness is thought to take up approximately 25 per cent of a GP's time. Mortality from coronary heart disease is falling but the number of deaths from suicide remains high, particularly among young men and this is a public health problem (Forth Valley Health Board 2000).

The number of frail elderly in nursing homes has swollen due to the closure of long-stay hospital beds. Individuals benefited as nursing homes may provide excellent care in environments much more pleasant than a hospital ward. Most GPs, however, have considerable experience of dealing with patients in this age group and there are great variations in care provided by nursing homes. In too many cases the medical care of these patients is barely adequate and there is a threat of sudden catastrophic closure of homes as a result of financial problems. This can hardly be the most secure way to provide care to the fast-growing population of frail elderly in the United Kingdom, but nevertheless the trend to offload the care of these patients to primary care continues (Drury 2001).

Hospital offloading happens in all medical fields and brings new challenges to the practice. Rising drug misuse, for example, has led to GPs being involved in substitute prescribing as well as managing a difficult and demanding patient group. Methadone prescribing in this way has led to the public health achievement of reducing the spread of AIDS in drug addicts (Wodak 1996). But not all GPs have been willing to share the burden with their secondary care colleagues. Some view drug abuse as primarily a social problem. New guidelines may help alter this view with workload distribution to be accompanied by resource distribution (Gabbay 2000). GPs are driven by financial realism and are not necessarily altruistic or realistic about the practicalities of care delivery.

The public health role of the GP: examples of good practice

Much of this chapter has been critical of GPs as profit-conscious practitioners who, though they may care for the individual, are narrow-minded. However, the average GP fulfils several useful public health functions in the following areas.

Infectious diseases

Public Health Departments in Health Boards rightly coordinate care in disease outbreaks, especially in very infectious illnesses affecting many patients in a practice or where a population spans many practices in a region. For example, during the *E. Coli* outbreak in Scotland in 1996, Public Health Consultants came to Health Centres to chair multi-disciplinary meetings involving all members of the PCT, bacteriologists, and hospital staff representatives. This communication is vital during any disease outbreak. Visits to Health Centres by Public Health Consultants are rare.

More commonly, a case of infectious disease, for example meningitis, is reported to the Public Health Department who then fax or e-mail all GPs in the region pertinent information on how to manage worried families, and advice on remaining vigilant for signs of further cases. The system seems to work well. It often involves out-of-hours communication with GPs and the development of GP out-of-hours cooperatives has also helped this communication. Whether NHS Direct will be useful in this context remains to be seen.

Media 'scares'

Media impacts are considerable and much health 'information' is incorrect or not peer-reviewed. For example, after the adverse publicity on the third generation combined oral contraceptives received in 1997, GP practices were immediately inundated with worried women who wished to stop taking such contraceptives. The effects of this on GP workload, often occurring before real evidence reached the GP, could be overwhelming. A large number of women also abandoned contraception altogether with a corresponding rise in the number of terminations of pregnancy.

Keeping abreast of media scares is important for GPs and cannot be easily achieved without effective communication from the local Public Health Consultant. Faxes from the local Consultant, or sometimes from the Chief Medical Officer, give the GP ammunition to face the onslaught when it comes. Patients, however, also now use the internet and may find 'information' which the Public Health Consultant is blissfully unaware of. The GPs then need to provide the patient with a balanced view of this information. This takes time and skill in critically appraising papers. Critical Appraisal is now part of the examination for the Royal College of General Practitioners (RCGP). This was not always the case and many older GPs do not hold this qualification.

The media may convey accurate health information to the population for instance regarding tobacco, diet, alcohol and exercise. Cot deaths declined following advice on sleeping position, supported by research, from a celebrity, whose own child had died of cot death. No Smoking Day and other initiatives rely heavily on the media to reach a wide population. If messages are correct and correctly remembered by the patient, the GP is there to reinforce the message. Populations do not always act on the information they receive. Smokers may ignore the health warnings on cigarettes. But the same message, coming from various sources, has a better chance of producing results. For this reason the proliferation of GPs writing in women's magazines, men's magazines and newspapers is to be welcomed.

Often there may be no evidence for many of the activities and treatments that are given in primary care. Thus, the GP and the patient have to live with the uncertainty about the effectiveness of interventions. GPs are generally quite used to coping with uncertainty although the patient may not be. GPs can communicate some of these dilemmas to the patient, and it is by a sharing of uncertainty that the ideal consultation should end with the patient and doctor making a joint decision on the future management (Elwyn *et al.* 2000).

Involvement in planning

Health Service developments are to be mediated by the use of Health Plans, which are agreed locally by committees including representatives from primary care, secondary care, public health, Health Board Administration and on occasion local council representatives. Users of the NHS have a role to play in planning, and public participation is to be a compulsory part of PCG functioning (Fisher and Gillam 2000). Primary care is the place where most citizens interface with the NHS and so it should have an extensive and invaluable role in the development of such programmes. This is often the case with GPs being invited to take part in most planning meetings which require some form of primary care input. These meetings are often chaired by Public Health Consultants or have input from this speciality. Few GPs usually have the time or inclination to attend such meetings and hence such events may not provide a balanced view to the committee. Other local Health Plan developments have all but ignored the view of the GPs who attend the meetings. In one case, the development of a guideline for local management of cancer services began after referral to hospital. The GP was present at earlier meetings but was not invited to subsequent ones.

GPs may also be too slow to come forward to attend such meetings, despite the offer of locum payments for those who attend. Yet, they must become involved as planning and budgeting are devolved down the administrative chain towards the PCTs. GPs have an important role in informing committees about practicalities involved in improving the health of practice populations although they will accept the expertise of Public Health Consultants when discussing issues such as needs assessment. Most GPs are unfamiliar with the concept of needs assessment. One study showed that there was no evidence that needs assessment had contributed to GP decisions regarding commissioning of care (Murie *et al.* 2000). If GPs do not become involved in planning, decisions will be taken without their input. Frustration may then occur at practice level if the plan is unpopular, or if the development of a plan is unworkable at grassroots level.

Screening

Screening the population has become a major part of the daily work of the GP. Screening ideally picks up disease at an early and more treatable stage. This benefits individual patients and from a public health viewpoint also provides value for money. It is cheaper to manage a well-controlled diabetic than wait for the same patient to have nephropathy before making the diagnosis of diabetes. There are national programmes which are well-developed such as child health surveillance, cervical smear programmes, breast mammography programme and more diseases are being diagnosed earlier.

This is good for the patients but creates three obvious problems. First, there is considerable patient anxiety created by some of the screening tests especially when awaiting results. This fuels the already rising tide of 'worried well' that fill the surgeries daily. There is an added issue of understanding that screening is not always needed – for example, explaining to a middle-aged man that he *doesn't* need his Prostate Specific Antigen (PSA) checked to look for prostate cancer. Describing the meaning of risk to patients is time-consuming. Second, the amount of screening activity is rising without a concomitant rise in GP numbers so that the service is gradually getting pushed to its limit. GPs are or soon will be involved in screening patients for diabetes, cancer of the colon, dementia, chlamydia, hypertension and obesity, and the list is likely to grow larger. Who in the PCT will undertake large targeted screening programmes? While the political will to reduce illnesses such as CHD appears to exist, no one has yet fully addressed the anxieties of the practitioners on the frontline (Evans 2000). Third, screening can become a mechanical activity with box ticking leading to the screening check being completed without the patient's wider problems being addressed. For example, child health surveillance, which like immunisation is now almost exclusively performed in GP surgeries by GPs and Health Visitors. This became an increasingly popular activity in primary care after the 1990 Contract, partly due to the financial incentives offered to GPs who would undertake this activity. Most children were being checked for developmental defects at intervals and computerised systems sprang up to recall the children at the right intervals. However, the third Hall Report subsequently argued that these checks were often unnecessary. Time could be better spent talking to the mothers about smoking, children's diet, behaviour management, dental care and so on. A major public health role for GPs and other members of the PCT was being missed, by concentrating on the 'check' rather than advising the family. Unfortunately the advice of the Hall Report has not been taken on board. If anything the paperwork now involved in performing the checks has left the patient even less likely to be advised on the above subjects (Hall 1996).

The formation in England of a National Screening Committee to provide advice across the whole gamut of possible screening programmes is an important advance. One of the first substantial products of that initiative has been a recommendation that screening for prostatic carcinoma should not be introduced (Scally 1998). Screening is an example of secondary prevention – picking up a disease and hopefully altering its course to prevent further deterioration. GPs also have a role in Primary Prevention – this is the process of changing patients' behaviour to prevent disease happening in the first place. Encouraging patients to stop smoking, drink in moderation and exercise more are daily occurrences in the GP's surgery. Collectively, GPs could help about half a million patients a year to stop smoking (Russell *et al.* 1979). Other members of the PCT such as Health Visitors are more active on this subject than GPs.

Immunisation

Immunisation programmes have radically reduced the incidence of many infectious diseases in the United Kingdom like measles, whooping cough, tetanus and diphtheria. This is a good example of successful primary prevention. Globally there have been many examples of re-emergence of disease when immunisation schedules are relaxed. Measles morbidity and mortality in Dublin rose when controversy over the safety of the MMR vaccine led to a fall in the number of immunised children. Public Health Departments coordinate immunisation activity for each region, and a complex communication method allows the Chief Medical Officer to keep GPs regularly informed of developments in this field.

Immunisation of babies and small children now happens almost exclusively in GPs' surgeries. There is, however, still a role for the school health service which has performed the mammoth tasks of MMR and meningococcal vaccination for school-age children in recent years. GPs have helped with catch-up campaigns. Vaccinations for travel abroad are now an area of expertise for many in primary care (particularly Practice Nurses), helped by internet-based information such as TRAVAX. Many occupations now recommend hepatitis B vaccination.

There is also the annual influenza vaccination programme which has now been expanded to include the over-65 age group. The influenza vaccination campaign illustrates how good information can lead to appropriate focussing of effort. GP surgeries are the only organisations that can coordinate the vaccination of the disparate at-risk groups: asthmatics, diabetics, those on immuno-suppressive therapy and so on.

Nevertheless infectious disease in the United Kingdom is still a major source of morbidity. There is evidence that TB is rising in incidence in certain vulnerable groups both in the United Kingdom and abroad. In addition drug resistant TB is rising. The need for continued, dedicated, organised programmes of immunisation is likely to remain an important pillar of the NHS's role in disease prevention. GPs will carry out the majority of immunisations separate from TB prevention work. Few GPs have the training to give the intradermal BCG injection, which is usually performed by the School Health Service or specially trained respiratory liaison nurses (Salisbury and Begg 1996).

Links

GPs have a very important public health role acting as a link in a chain of communication between agencies. When guidelines on prevention of coronary heart disease for instance are published by a national organisation, local GP surgeries will put the advice into practice. This may be through starting smoking cessation clinics, checking patients' cholesterol levels, employing nurses, and altering prescribing to allow for findings of new research. When breast screening by mammography is organised in a region, GP practices check patients' addresses, advertise and encourage the uptake of the screening service.

GPs link with many agencies in the NHS and with pharmacists, social work departments, employers and voluntary groups. They are often 'ideally placed' to coordinate, for example, the care of the mentally handicapped in the community. One other relevant link, often forgotten is with drug companies who besiege GP surgeries because the vast majority of drugs taken by patients in the United Kingdom are prescribed by their GP with the exception of medications available over the counter from pharmacists. Drug companies led major improvements in the health of certain populations. For example, in the 1980s in asthma care with GPs prescribing more preventative steroid inhalers. Drug companies developed asthma courses for nurses, vast amounts of patient literature and encouraged the prescribing of steroid inhalers. Subsequently the control of asthma patients has improved and drug companies can take some of the credit. As the management of other diseases alters, drug companies have produced cholesterol-testing kits and osteoporosis audits. These boost their sales and in instances where there is a sound evidence base they have improved patient health.

GPs provide a direct link to their local public health department by reporting cases of infectious disease although this is a variable service. Some GPs report all cases and others only remember to do so on occasion. Food poisoning is an example. 'What is the prevalence of food poisoning in the community?' cannot be answered by asking the clinicians who most frequently deal with the condition. Most patients with diarrhoea will have no contact with the NHS and perhaps visit their pharmacist. Most patients who see their GP do not have stool samples tested by GPs. The local lab may not test for self-limiting conditions such as *B. Cereus* or *Clos. Difficile* so that a normal result from the lab does not mean that food poisoning is excluded. Although a fee is paid to GPs for reporting each case, on this occasion the financial carrot does not appear to be enough to encourage GPs to report every case seen. Until this happens, health needs assessments will be incomplete.

Partnership with other agencies such as local councils is becoming more common with the development of Healthy Living Centres and other initiatives which involve the local community. As most of the NHS effort is directed towards established disease, these attempts to switch to more preventive community medicine are welcome. This is partly due to publications of influential reports such as 'Towards a Healthier Scotland' which emphasise multi-agency working in which GPs must play their part.

Link establishment should involve the GPs at the beginning to be successful otherwise GPs may be suspicious of the usefulness of the service being provided. NHS Direct faced initial opposition from many GPs because it was developed rapidly and with little GP consultation. NHS Direct needs to reach the people who find it hardest to gain access to health services but has had problems publicising itself and has not targeted the most vulnerable in our communities. This could become another example of the Inverse Care Law. If properly developed, however, NHS Direct has the potential to bring an equal standard of health advice to people across the country (Pearce and Rosen 2000).

Consultations

GPs in some respects carry out public health work in many individual consultations. The consultation, although with an individual, locates the patient in their family and community setting. Broader issues such as income, chances of employment and housing can have a bearing on the consultation and may be the underlying reason why the patient has made an appointment in the first place. Each individual consultation should ideally consist of a detailed analysis of the patient's problems, diagnosis with or without investigation, advice and treatment, opportunistic screening if appropriate, followed by health education backed up with an advice leaflet. Of course this is not achievable in every case as the average consultation in Scotland lasts only six minutes. The screening, Health Education and advice leaflet are often left out of the consultation.

Studies have shown that longer consultations – ten minutes per patient – allow GPs to pick up more psychological problems.

Advice from the RCGP in 2000 is encouraging all GPs to adopt a longer consultation of ten minutes per patient. This can only lead to better care, with the added bonus that some of the Our Healthier Nation targets may be better addressed (RCGP 2000).

Working together

This is rather revolutionary for most GPs. Despite disagreements between local practices about how to manage each problem, the formation of Localities and LHCCs/Primary Care Groups will gradually lead to more effective management of larger populations of patients. The formation of these groups was made easier by their coincidental formation of 'on call cooperatives' which drew practices together into on-call organisations, some of which include over 100 GPs working together to care for whole cities or counties out-of-hours. By spending long hours at weekends and overnight together, GPs have been able to overcome barriers between practices, paving the way for group work at the LHCC/PCT level by day.

This activity had significant public health repercussions because these groups of GPs began to standardise care for certain conditions, collect supplies of relevant emergency medicine and go on courses to improve defibrillation skills. Also, if the local public health department wishes to contact a large number of GPs at a weekend, it is easier to contact a single out-of-hours cooperative, than try to contact 70 different practices who previously would have worked independently.

Conclusions – looking to the future

The Inverse Care Law

Those with the greatest health needs are most vulnerable. They are less likely to know where to get reliable health information and least likely to take advice when they receive it. They live in the poorest areas of the United Kingdom and the gap between the richest and the poorest appears to be widening. As the richer members of our society get more access to private health care, eat better diets, smoke less, breastfeed more and so on, the poorer members do the opposite. It could be argued that some of the major threats to our health in the West such as poverty, obesity, smoking, drug addiction, alcohol abuse and pollution are beyond the control of the Health Service or indeed any service. The inequalities in health in the United Kingdom continue to exist at the beginning of the twenty-first century, despite the link between poverty and health being commented on and researched for over 150 years. Health inequalities have, shamefully, lost their power to shock (Pownall 1999a).

Should GPs be involved in improving health care, or should they instead concentrate on improving income distribution, education, nutrition and physical environments? (Sram and Ashton 1998). They have a responsibility to do all these things, in their role as the patients' advocate. GPs spend some of their time when they are not seeing patients referring them to appropriate agencies, advising on housing and other social issues, and liaising with employers. Their role has changed over the years and become more active, instead of passively waiting for the ill patient to appear in the surgery although this is still the largest part of their workload.

GPs are acutely aware that those who do the greatest amount of 'caring' are not financially rewarded for doing so. Primary care is less well resourced than secondary care, although most of the 'care' occurs away from the consultants' hospital clinic. GPs working in the poorest areas find their workload greater than their colleagues who work in leafy suburbs or rural practices. Their patients develop multiple pathologies due to adverse lifestyle and patient problem lists may be expanded by domestic abuse, drug abuse, workplace accidents and many other conditions which may be rarer entities for the suburban GP. With higher consultation rates in poorer areas, the GP becomes more exhausted more quickly and has less time for the vital health education and screening role. These are all major public health issues.

As the United Kingdom becomes more multi-cultural, training of GPs needs to take into account the different needs of ethnic groups. Health inequalities exist between various ethnic groups in our society, for example, with differences in the rates of ischaemic heart disease, diabetes and smoking. To address these health problems, GPs need to be aware of the different health-seeking behaviours of different groups and reach out to those groups who

are at present not receiving care needed or accessing health promotion material (DoH 1999). There are a growing number of
homeless people who are often not registered with a GP, who have
significant physical and mental health problems, representing an
unmet need in our affluent society. Providing primary care services to the growing group of refugees and asylum seekers in the
United Kingdom and throughout the world is an important public
health issue. As these vulnerable people often come from areas of
war and famine, they may have many psychological problems and
acute or chronic infectious illnesses including malaria, hepatitis B
and C and drug-resistant tuberculosis. They may not gain access to
health maintenance programmes and therefore may be incorrectly
or inadequately immunised (Hargreaves *et al.* 2000).

Resources

As data from primary care becomes more complete, with initiatives
like the Practice Development Plan and Continuous Morbidity
Recording, the full picture of the effect that disease has on the
population becomes clearer. Hard-pressed GPs are hopeful
that this will also lead to more resource being fed to areas of
greatest need.

The shift of control of budgets downwards, from central government to health boards, subsequently to PCTs, helps the local
GPs have a say in what is being spent in their area. Few GPs, however, have any grasp of health economics. They may make daily
individual decisions about funding in their own surgeries but not
all have the ability to see the bigger financial picture while serving
on, for example, a PCT Drug Budget Committee covering a whole
region. There is also a danger of creating a 'postcode lottery'. Care
must be taken that the country does not become divided, as in the
1980s and 1990s, into those practices which were fundholders, and
those which were not. Most benefits of commissioning relate to
improved professional relationships, not to service changes. Locality
commissioning does not appear to have resulted in major changes
to contracts or services (Hudson Hart *et al.* 1999).

The NHS funding increase in 2000 apparently aimed to be more
focussed towards the areas of greatest need, with a particular
emphasis on deprived areas with initiatives such as Social Inclusion

Partnerships. If this is more than government rhetoric, it is a very welcome news, and could herald the beginning of the end of the Inverse Care Law. However, some of the information used to make recommendations such as the Arbuthnott Report may have been incomplete with the result that there is a need for further research to provide better estimates of the need for health care (Watt 1999).

Recruitment

Since the 1990 New Contract the number of applicants to GP training schemes has fallen dramatically because of rises in workload and administration, and a sense that GPs are losing their autonomy. This is particularly true in deprived areas, where the workload is so great that there is less time to perform some of the preventative care discussed in this chapter. In addition, on call commitment for many hospital doctors becomes easier as they grow more senior, while a GP's commitment is likely to stay constant despite increasing age. Junior doctors are showing less interest in General Practice, insufficient numbers of GPs are being trained, a large cohort of GPs are nearing retirement, and the numbers of consultants is to be expanded. There will soon be a large deficit in the number of GPs available, and this calls into question whether some of the above public health activities will be fitted into the busy workload of those who remain (RCGP 1999).

It is also a worry that GPs, when trained and looking for a practice, are more attracted to the rural or more affluent areas though single-handed remote practices, in the Scottish Highlands for example, also have recruitment problems. The most important influence on a GP's choice of practice is aversion to working in an area of high deprivation (Gosden *et al.* 2000). As the numbers of applicants to poorer areas falls, the overall quality of applicants to work in these areas also falls. There are of course many exceptions, with many dedicated GPs performing excellent work in 'difficult' areas, but the fact remains that recruitment of GPs to all areas, affluent or not, is a problem. This has serious repercussions for the Public Health Agenda – who will carry out the work in the areas that need it most?

Incentives to encourage GPs to work for the poorer areas of the United Kingdom have been brought in to try and reverse the Inverse Care Law. On-call arrangements such as the development of out-of-hours cooperatives are showing that a lifelong on-call commitment can be coped with by innovation. The development of Personal Medical Services was partly brought about by the need to serve poorer populations better. The availability of an extended primary care team, and the ability to develop outside interests, have been suggested as other ways to attract GPs into currently under-served areas (Pownall 1999b).

Education and reform

> There is nothing more difficult to carry out, nor more doubtful of success, nor more dangerous to handle, than to initiate a new order of things. (Machiavelli)

The NHS is tired of reform but reform continues and there is still a need for changes to tackle the problems outlined in this chapter. The rise in the profile of evidence-based medicine has encouraged many GPs to look again at their work and their role within practice and PCTs. Other members of the team now perform many tasks which GPs did in the past. The GP's role now is partly co-coordinator of services for local populations. However, there is a lack of evidence about the public health role of GPs. They also have little training in public health – no more than a few lectures as a medical student, and some instruction on the basics of epidemiology as a GP Registrar. Thereafter education is a mixed bag and public health takes a lowly position beside clinical skills, pharmacology, disease management and so on. Many GPs are unable to provide any information on their public health role apart from perhaps the immunisation or smear target that they have achieved. There is a need for greater and regular liaison between GPs and their local public health departments.

In the closing years of the twentieth century a number of initiatives were set up in the United Kingdom to encourage research in primary care. This involved the setting up of primary care research networks which have established themselves as a useful laboratory for the study of diseases in populations, although their usefulness is yet to be fully evaluated (Clement 2000). Most of the research during the last 50 years has taken place in the hospital setting but those patients who reach secondary care are not at all representative of the population as a whole. The information which will come from this new emphasis on primary care research will be more generalisable and lead to a greater understanding of the disease processes in the community. It will also encourage a culture of research in primary care, with subsequent increased awareness of the need to solve previously 'insoluble' problems, such as frequent attenders in GP surgeries.

Clinical governance

As patients become more aware of illness via the media and the Internet, the role of the GP is changing. GPs are no longer the sole holders of information who inform the patient exclusively. Now GPs filter the information for the patient. This change has led to more GPs becoming familiar with critical appraisal of literature. A well-informed population is to be encouraged. As patients become 'informed', the need for a better-informed GP has never been greater as a result. GPs are able to access high quality information via the NHS net. The revalidation of all GPs will encourage all GPs to do this and, though revalidation has critics, it will lead to a better health service for all.

The education of GPs, the rise in the profile of evidence-based medicine, audit and focussing of services based on need, are all part of the concept called Clinical Governance. GP education is changing with more focus on evidence-based medicine and narrowing the gap between research and practice. The old method of Postgraduate Education for GPs, usually involving attendance at several lectures throughout the year, has been criticised and may now be shortly abolished. The system was too passive, static and not led by individual needs. Instead a more active mode of education, with the personal learning plan becoming widespread, and led by the needs of the individual practitioner or practice, has been suggested.

This process should lead to GPs avoiding the old pitfalls such as the rush for Health Promotion payments described earlier and a more patient-centred NHS should emerge. Few GPs admit to not being patient-centred. The topic has much momentum and may bring about changes that improve the health of the patients but do not make GPs lives easier. The NHS is at times set up with the needs of the professionals too high on the agenda. Men's health is a good example of a problem area with men dying younger than women, attending health checks less often, committing suicide and living less healthy lifestyles generally. Yet, many men rightly claim that they cannot see their GP easily due to work pressures. The suggested answer is to encourage GPs to have surgeries in the evenings and at weekends. This is likely to be unpopular with GPs, but is a patient-centred answer to the problem (SEHD 2001).

Organisations such as the RCGP have long campaigned to improve overall quality in general practice. Practice Accreditation, and Quality Practice Awards, both organised by the RCGP, are encouraging GPs to have built-in practice systems for looking at preventive health services, health promotion, chronic disease care, mental health services and other areas, which have a clear public health benefit. There is, however, a need to be realistic about what can be achieved with an already overstretched workforce. Although the GP is often described as 'ideally placed' to deal with major public health concerns such as obesity, alcohol abuse, smoking and hypertension screening (RCGP 1991), there are only limited resources, particularly time, for the average GP to spend on these activities.

'Why is it every time that I mention the word "reform" GPs reach nervously for their wallets?' Kenneth Clarke, former secretary of state for health, was partly right. Most UK general practices are small businesses, understandably influenced by financial incentives and disincentives or 'the imagination, enterprise and investment assumptions of corner shopkeeping' (Foy *et al.* 1998). To change the way a practice works either for profit or for the good of the practice population takes energy and ability, which not all GPs possess.

At the beginning of the twenty-first century a 'new' GP Contract is being negotiated with the profession which may bring some important public health benefits. GPs will be rewarded for quality care, which they will need to prove according to an evidence base, in vulnerable groups such as diabetics and those with coronary heart disease. The method of payment will encourage this 'quality' care, and move away from the number-crunching of previous payment systems. This, allied to the annual appraisal of individual GPs, will gradually lead to less variation in quality of care across the population.

Few GPs are aware of the incidence of illness in their locality, and are ill-equipped and not sufficiently trained to do anything about this. They need lifelong training in the relevance and management of public health issues. Research has shown some cynicism in the UK GPs, some of whom are reluctant to take a population approach to lifestyle advice and remain unconvinced about the effectiveness of their intervention (Lawlor *et al.* 2000). Grateful patients are few in the field of preventive medicine where success is a 'non-event'. As GPs' time is limited, public health may not be a priority. Financial incentives may be needed to encourage GPs otherwise. Rewarding doctors for activities that prevent ill health is an issue that has not been solved in the United Kingdom or elsewhere (Rose 1992).

Plus ça change, plus c'est le même chose.

References

Baker R (2001) Is it time to review the idea of compliance with guidelines? *Br J Gen Pract* **51**: 7–9.

Clement S (2000) Towards a conceptual framework for evaluating primary care research networks. *Br J Gen Pract* **50**: 651–3.

DOH (1999) *Health Survey for England 'New Survey Highlights Health Inequalities Among Ethnic Groups'.* Department of Health, London.

Drury M (2001) Aging Britain – challenges and opportunities for general practice. *Br J Gen Pract* **51**: 5–7.

Elwyn G *et al.* (2000) Shared decision-making in primary care: the neglected second half of the consultation. *Br J Gen Pract* **49**: 477–83.

Evans P (2000) The primary prevention of CHD with statins: practice headache or public health? *Br J Gen Pract* **50**: 695–7.

Fisher B and Gillam S (2000) Community development in the new NHS. *Br J Gen Pract* **49**: 428–31.

Forth Valley Health Board (2000) *The Health of the Population of Forth Valley 1999–2000.* FVHB, Stirling, pp 15–17.

Foy R, Parry J and McAvoy B (1998) Clinical trials in primary care. *BMJ* **317**: 1168–9.

Gabbay M (2000) A cautious welcome for the new guidelines on management of drug dependence. *Br J Gen Pract* **50**: 91–2.

Gosden T, Bowler I and Sutton M (2000) How do GPs choose their practice? Estimating the strength of GP preferences for practice and job characteristics. *J Health Serv Res Pol* **5**(4): 208–13.

Hall D (1996) *Health for all Children*, 3rd edn. Oxford University Press, Oxford, pp 36–7.

Hargreaves S *et al.* (2000) Refugees, asylum seekers and general practice: room for improvement. *Br J Gen Pract* **50**: 531–2.

Hudson Hart C *et al.* (1999) Locality commissioning: how much influence have GPs really had? *Br J Gen Pract* **49**: 903–5.

Koperski M (2000) The state of primary care in the USA and lessons for primary care groups in the UK. *Br J Gen Pract* **50**: 319–23.

Lawlor S *et al.* (2000) Can GPs influence the nation's health through a population approach to provision of lifestyle advice? *Br J Gen Pract* **50**: 455–60.

Lough J *et al.* (2000) Supporting practice-based audit: a price to be paid for collecting data. *Br J Gen Pract* **49**: 793–6.

Murie J *et al.* (2000) Needs assessment in primary care: GPs' perceptions and implications for the future. *Br J Gen Pract* **50**: 17–21.

Pearce K and Rosen R (2000) NHS Direct. King's Fund, London, p 38.

Pownall M (1999a) Poor need access to more cash. *Medical Interface* 8–12 March.

Pownall M (1999b) PMS pilots will help GPs break free from Red Book strictures. *Prim Care Rep* **1**(4): 8.

RCGP (1991) Preventive Medicine, pp 20, 35, 50, 65.

RCGP (1999) Practice Development – Quality Team.

RCGP (2000) Valuing Scottish General Practice, pp 8–9.

Rose G (1992) *The Strategy of Preventive Medicine*. Oxford University Press, Oxford, pp 105–6.

Russell MAH *et al.* (1979) Effects of General Practitioners advice against smoking. *BMJ* **2**: 31.

Salisbury DM and Begg NT (eds) (1996) *Immunisation Against Infectious Disease*. Department of Health and Others, HMSO, London. pp 221–5.

Scally G (1998) Recent advances, Public Health (Clinical Review). *BMJ* **317**(47): 584–6.

SEHD (Scottish Executive Health Department) (2001) *Our National Health, A Plan for Action, A Plan for Change*. SEHD, Edinburgh.

Sram I and Ashton J (1998) Millennium report to Sir Edwin Chadwick. *BMJ* **317**: 592–6.

Starfield B (2001) New paradigms for quality in Primary Care. *Br J Gen Pract* **51**: 303–11.

Watt G (1999) After Arbuthnott: many questions still need to be asked. *The magazine of RCGP (Scotland)* **24**: 4–5.

WHO Collaborative Group (1998) *WHO Phase 111 Collaborative Study on Implementing and Supporting Early Intervention Strategies in Primary Health Care*. WHO, Copenhagen.

Wodak A (1996) A stupendous public health achievement. *Addiction* **8**: 1090–2.

7

Housing and Health

Isobel Anderson and Aileen Barclay

Introduction

Housing, health and well-being have always been inextricably linked. Shelter is a basic life necessity and adequate, affordable housing, in a secure neighbourhood, is commonly taken to be a fundamental prerequisite for healthy and happy living. Arguably, the broad principle that adequate housing is essential to public health offers as strong a case for positive state intervention in the housing system as do housing-specific objectives. Similarly, the varied input of the housing profession into providing and managing housing, and to supporting the well-being of tenants and residents, contributes in no small measure to public health outcomes as well as housing outcomes. Consequently, an understanding of the operation of the housing system and contribution of the housing profession will be essential to any comprehensive analysis of public health.

The aim of this chapter is to provide an insight into contemporary housing provision in the United Kingdom and to discuss the implications for public health and well-being. The discussion is not exhaustive, but sets out the key issues and points to sources of further information. The first section presents an overview of the state of the UK housing stock at the start of the twenty-first century, and highlights the key determinants of change. The research evidence on the links between housing and health is then examined. Next, the chapter sets out the most recent policy changes in housing under the post-1997 New Labour governments, highlighting links with public health and well-being. Recommended good practice for housing and health interventions is then examined, prior to drawing conclusions on current issues for housing and public health.

Housing in the United Kingdom

In contrast to health care and other dimensions of welfare (e.g. education), most of the UK's housing stock is provided through the market or private sector, rather than being directly delivered through the welfare state. That is to say, most households secure their housing by renting or buying it in the market place. Historically, this has always been the case. Only in Scotland, for a relatively short period in the second half of the twentieth century, did public sector housing account for more than 50 per cent of the total dwelling stock (O'Carroll 1996: p 17, Table 2.1).

Moreover, the notions of 'public' and 'private' provision are not straightforward in housing. Private sector tenants on low incomes can receive state assistance through housing benefit. For much of the twentieth century, home owners received significant state subsidies through mortgage interest tax relief, although this was gradually phased out under New Labour and has now been abolished. Similarly, the 'voluntary' sector has benefited significantly from government funded capital and revenue grants. For example, since the late 1980s, housing associations have been funded through a mix of private and public monies.

Determining local and national housing requirements is highly complex. Demand for housing results from a combination of household formation/change, demographic trends, changes in the economy/labour market and social/cultural trends (Anderson 1994). Housing supply, provided through the market and social sectors, is usually expected to last a minimum of 30 years and much of the dwelling stock is significantly older. Given that housing cannot be quickly produced or readily moved around, supply is not highly responsive to changes in demand. The system is subject to a mismatch between supply and demand in terms of location, type, quality and cost. These characteristics of the housing system present significant challenges for governments and housing providers trying to meet housing needs as a key element of well-being.

During the twentieth century, the United Kingdom experienced a massive transformation in housing tenure (Malpass and Murie 1999). At the beginning of the century, more than 90 per cent of the dwelling stock was in the privately rented sector. The poor housing conditions associated with rapid urbanisation and industrialisation led to state intervention early in the twentieth century, largely driven by concerns about public health (notably contagious diseases, such as cholera, which largely resulted from poor sanitation). At that time, central government saw local authorities as the obvious vehicle for the provision of state subsidised housing and council housing came into being. The period up to the end of the 1970s saw sustained growth in council housing along with the rapid expansion of home ownership. Private renting had been reduced to a minor tenure, accounting for less than 10 per cent of the housing stock by the 1980s.

These changes in housing tenure patterns were largely explained by a combination of factors, associated with changes in policy and practice across the twentieth century:

• Local authority new housebuilding for rent (and to a much lesser extent, voluntary sector housing association new build and refurbishment).
• The increased availability of mortgage finance for home ownership through building societies and banks, combined with tax relief on interest paid on home loans.
• The development of new housing for sale to individual households, by speculative housebuilders.
• The demolition of privately rented dwellings in poor condition through slum clearance programmes (largely replaced by council housing).
• The transfer of privately rented dwellings into home ownership through individual sales by landlords (associated with the decline in profitability of private renting due to tighter regulation and financial incentives for home ownership).

Of these factors, slum clearance programmes and the expansion of council housing (up until the late 1970s) contributed significantly to improvements in public health.

By the late twentieth century new trends in housing tenure had become established, despite some variation within the United

Kingdom (Table 7.1). Home ownership had become the dominant tenure across the United Kingdom and public renting was already beginning to decline. From 1980, council housing began to decline due to increased sales to sitting tenants, under the 'Right to Buy', combined with cuts in investment in new council housing. In later years, this continuing lack of new public investment in council housing was a key driver for larger scale transfer of local authority housing stock to housing associations or new types of social landlords (Murie and Nevin 2001; Mullen 2001).

The housing association sector more than doubled in scale between 1981 and 1998, though it still comprised less than 5 per cent

Table 7.1 Housing tenure in the United Kingdom: 1981–98

Housing tenure as % of total housing stock	Home ownership (%)	Privately rented (%)	Housing Association/ RSL[1] rented (%)	Council/ NIHE[2] rented (%)	Total (%)
Scotland					
1981	36.4	9.7	1.8	52.2	100
1998[3]	61.3	6.7	5.3	26.6	100
England					
1981	58.2	11.3	2.3	28.1	100
1998	68.0	11.1	5.0	15.9	100
Wales					
1981	62.6	9.4	1.1	26.9	100
1998	71.5	8.5	4.0	16.0	100
Northern Ireland					
1981	54.0	7.6	1.1	37.9	100
1998	71.3	4.4	2.5	22.0	100
United Kingdom					
1981	56.4	11.0	2.2	30.4	100
1998	67.6	10.4	4.9	17.0	100

Notes

[1] RSL: Registered Social Landlord. This term embraces both housing associations and other types of landlord registered with the relevant bodies across the UK and eligible to receive government funded subsidy for the building, refurbishment and management of social oriented housing.

[2] NIHE: Northern Ireland Housing Executive, main provider of public rented housing in Northern Ireland.

[3] 1998 was the most recent year for which figures were available at the time of writing.

Source: Adapted from Wilcox (2000), Table 17b, p 103 and Table 17d, p 105.

of the total housing stock. Expansion was brought about through new housebuilding, combined with the more recent trend of housing associations and other 'registered social landlords' taking over the ownership of former council housing. The decline in the council rented sector is evident from Table 7.1. In Scotland, council housing was the majority tenure in 1981, but accounted for just over one-quarter of the housing stock by 1998. For England and Wales, the proportion of the housing stock in the council sector declined from just over a quarter to less than one-fifth, with Northern Ireland having just around one-fifth of all housing in the public sector. Nevertheless, local authority housing remained the main provider of affordable rented housing, albeit in a state of considerable flux.

Legal standards for housing (covering space, state of repair, provision of sanitation and so on) also evolved during the twentieth century. By 2000, only a very small proportion of households in the United Kingdom (6 per cent) lived in dwellings classified as unfit for human habitation or below the Scottish tolerable standard (Revell and Leather 2000). Geographically, the most problematic areas were South Wales, rural Wales and Scotland, industrial districts of the north of England and some cities in the Midlands. Disrepair was more of a problem than unfitness, with almost one-third of homes in England needing repairs costing more than £1000 and 30 per cent of those in Scotland needing work costing more than £3000 (Revell and Leather 2000). Some households are more likely to live in dwellings in a poor state of repair than others. Disrepair is highest in the private rented sector and among older dwellings, with converted flats and terraces most likely to be in poor condition. Further, the poorest households suffer disproportionately from bad housing conditions. People on low incomes are nearly twice as likely to live in unfit housing as those on higher incomes and older people, along with those establishing their first home are also among those most likely to live in poor conditions (Revell and Leather 2000).

Under the New Right Conservative governments of 1979–97 strategies sought to reduce state intervention and public expenditure. The key focus of housing policy was the expansion of home ownership and public expenditure on housing was cut more severely than any other aspect of welfare (Wilcox 2000). Public subsidy was switched from 'bricks and mortar' (providing cheap homes) to 'people' (through Housing Benefit to assist low-income households pay higher rents). During the same period, vacant council housing was increasingly allocated to households deemed to be in the greatest need (e.g. overcrowded, lacking basic amenities and experiencing health problems). Gradually, lower income and economically inactive households became increasingly concentrated in the council and housing association sectors. Combined with sustained 'disinvestment' in the fabric of the housing stock, the result was a notable deterioration in the quality of life prevailing in the social housing sector, as compared to that of the 1960s and 1970s. Different types of housing-related public health issues began to emerge, as discussed below.

According to Kemp (1999), in some ways, Britain was better housed in 1997, compared to 1979. The proportion of households living in dwellings that lacked basic amenities or central heating had fallen and the overall state of repair of the housing stock improved in the 1980s. On the other hand, space standards in new rented housing were lowered and there was a £10 billion repair backlog in the council sector. There were also other ways in which the housing situation had deteriorated. The number of households accepted as homeless by local authorities doubled during the 1980s (Greve and Currie 1990) and remained at a high level throughout the 1990s. A combination of economic restructuring, market failure, cuts in social security benefits and exclusion from the homelessness safety net precipitated a street homelessness crisis in the late 1980s, of a magnitude which had never before been seen in Britain (Anderson 1993). Even the dream of home ownership turned into negative equity or repossession for many on the margins of this tenure (Ford 1993; Nettleton and Burrows 2000).

These were the housing circumstances which faced the New Labour government which came to power in 1997. The fit (or lack of fit) between housing supply and demand became increasingly differentiated across the country with intense pressure in the South East of England contrasting with oversupply and even 'abandonment' of housing in some parts of the North of England and Scotland (Lowe 2000). While most of the nation was well housed, sustained inequalities in access to housing and other aspects of welfare for those on the margins continued to raise complex challenges for housing provision (Anderson and Sim 2000).

Housing and health: making the links

Before looking at contemporary policy and practice on housing and health, it is important to consider the available evidence on the links between the two aspects of well-being. There is a significant body of research evidence on the links between health and housing and a number of authors have conducted detailed reviews (Universities of Sussex and Westminster 1996; Wilkinson 1999; Dunn 2000). The relationships between housing and health can be examined from two directions. Poor quality housing or being homeless is likely to have an impact on both physical and mental health and on the well-being of people with disabilities. Similarly, poor physical or mental health, or disability, may also constrain households' opportunities to gain access to their preferred or ideal housing. Housing itself can be considered in terms of both individual dwellings and in relation to the wider local environment or neighbourhood. In practice, these sets of relationships are likely to overlap and the interlinkages are likely to be complex. As other chapters in this book focus on varying dimensions of health and well-being, the remainder of this section is structured around 'housing dimensions' (neighbourhood, dwelling, care and support, and homelessness) with the links to public health issues being explored in relation to these housing factors.

Health and the neighbourhood

Although the individual dwelling might seem the most obvious focus for the links between housing and health, beginning the analysis with a consideration of the environment facilitates a systematic progression from the macro to the micro level of analysis. In a large-scale quantitative survey of the psycho-social benefits of home, neighbourhood context was found to have significant influence in relation to households' experience of home as a haven, locus of autonomy and source of status (Kearns *et al.* 2000).

Much previous research on housing and health has focussed on the physical environment in relation to physical health. There are well documented links between the existence of toxic substances in the built environment and related health problems. Examples include asbestos, radon gas and lead pipes (Wilkinson 1999). Exposure to asbestos dust can result in asbestos-related diseases years later, while radon gas (which can penetrate homes from the underlying rock structure) can cause lung cancer. The causes and consequences of these environmental hazards are well established, allowing appropriate remedial action to be taken.

The social and psychological impact of the residential environment on health has received increasing attention from researchers (Chartered Institute of Housing 1998; Ellaway *et al.* 1999). To some extent, this will be determined by a combination of the expectations of households and their lived experience in relation to the quality of the local environment. For example, families with young children who live in high rise blocks of flats, with no access to suitable play areas may suffer associated stress and constraints on child development. Quality in property management (e.g. maintenance of lifts) would be another influence. Much would depend, however, on the appropriateness of the dwelling for the household, as many better off households live quite satisfactorily in high quality, well maintained high rise buildings which suit their household type or preference.

The physical environment is increasingly recognised as a key link to mental health issues in particular. While individual dwellings may be perfectly sound in physical terms, the neighbourhood may be considered to be totally inappropriate. Unpopular areas may be associated with crime and the fear of crime, with noise, vandalism, theft/burglary, violence, harassment (including racism) and other types of nuisance (Chartered Institute of Housing 1998). These factors may cause considerable emotional stress leading to anxiety or depression and more serious health consequences such as physical assault. The local neighbourhood may also have an influence on access to health care in terms of the quality of local services and the availability of local resources and services. There may be related issues around public transport to health facilities, for example, from peripheral housing estates or rural locations.

In the above circumstances, housing and health disadvantage are likely to link to a more general experience of area based poverty/disadvantage across a range of indicators, such as education, employment and so on. Consequently, it is often difficult to isolate the impact of poor housing from other factors. Recent research has attempted to tackle this problem by developing a longitudinal analysis of the impact of housing deprivation on health (Marsh *et al.* 2000). The index of multiple deprivation goes beyond traditional concerns with the quality and amenity of a dwelling to incorporate key subjective factors such as satisfaction with dwelling or residential area. Multiple housing deprivation led to an average 25 per cent greater risk of disability or severe ill health across the life course (Marsh *et al.* 2000: p 425). The experience of both current and past poor housing was found to be significantly associated with greater likelihood of ill-health. Housing deprivation in early life influenced poor health in later life, even when housing circumstances improved.

Recent evidence on the impact of area regeneration is available from a study of two housing estates in Tower Hamlets where the health of residents was monitored as they were moved from run down housing into new properties (*Guardian* 2000). Residents reported significantly fewer days feeling ill and health improvements linked with less overcrowding, and fewer problems with dampness and infestations. It was acknowledged that not all of the identified health improvement was down to housing improvements, as there were other linked initiatives taking place simultaneously. However, it was also recognised that the process was disruptive. In this case, the area regeneration was linked to a change of landlord away from the local authority to a housing association and some disquiet was reported in relation to this and associated rent increases (*Guardian* 2000).

Arguably, extensive evidence now points fairly conclusively to a direct causal relationship between housing deprivation and the risk of ill-health (Marsh *et al.* 2000). In addition, significant improvements to health and quality of life for children and adults alike, resulting from housing investment in the course of urban regeneration have been documented (Ellaway *et al.* 1999). Consequently, the impact of housing policy and the work of housing professionals at the neighbourhood level, has both direct and indirect consequences for public health. Most directly, investment programmes bring about physical improvements to the quality of dwellings and the environment which will be beneficial to public health. However, in partnership with other agencies, the input of housing professionals into community initiatives can also have a significant impact in terms of combating problems such as crime and nuisance, resulting in safer, more secure neighbourhoods and improved psychological well-being.

Health and the individual dwelling

As with the neighbourhood level of analysis, the most evident and longest established links between health and the individual dwelling have related to the negative consequences of poor physical conditions for physical health. For example, there is a quite significant body of evidence on the impact of cold, damp housing on physical health. As well as being generally unpleasant, dampness and mould growth have been linked to asthma and other respiratory diseases, particularly in relation to children's health (Wilkinson 1999). The health impact of cold and damp housing can be exacerbated by climatic variation. Scotland experiences increased mortality in colder winters, raising issues around the effectiveness of heating and insulation. The installation of central heating has been shown to reduce respiratory problems and time off school for children, indicating the practical health benefits of straightforward improvements in housing (Wilkinson 1999).

As discussed above, large-scale urban renewal has been a key mechanism for improving housing conditions, especially in the public sector. However, a detailed study of the impact of the process of renewal for individual households suggests that the upheaval can cause considerable stress on some households, before long-term benefits are felt (Allen 2000). Refurbishment may be 'uninvited' on the part of tenants, who may lack any personal control of the process. During the process of renewal, some residents in the study experienced adverse health effects, while others did not. The issue of personal control, which was more important to some households than others, emerged as an explanatory factor. The nature of landlord/tenant relationships has changed in recent years as the argument that tenants should have more say in the management of their homes has gained widespread acceptance (Cooper and Hawtin 1998). The greater involvement of residents in the renewal process, which is now being embraced by the housing profession, could result in improved public health outcomes, as well as better tenant satisfaction with the refurbishment of their homes.

The physical design and layout of a dwelling are particularly important where a household member has a physical disability or limited mobility. Well designed, appropriate housing can make life much easier for someone with limited mobility while unsuitable housing can make life very difficult, resulting in worsening physical and mental health. However, the growth of the disability movement and the associated unwillingness to medicalise disability has contributed to the omission of disability-related issues from research on health and housing (Oldman and Beresford 2000). In contrast, the adverse effects on physical and mental health of unsuitable housing were reported, unprompted, by participants in a study of families where children had disabilities. Evidently, measures of housing deprivation need to be redefined to take account of circumstances which impact upon disability, but are not traditionally recognised as poor housing (Oldman and Beresford 2000).

As mentioned above, social rented housing is one sector of the system which has explicitly used health criteria for selection. While not an exclusive goal, selection in favour of sick and disabled people, with the intention of improving their health/well-being has been a key element of housing allocation policies (Smith *et al.* 1998). Medical rehousing has been found to be an effective health intervention, associated with moves into healthier housing, reduced symptoms and reduced demands on health care, though outcomes have been constrained by the limited capacity of a shrinking public sector to respond to needs or accommodate growing demand (Smith *et al.* 1998).

Research has only recently begun to ask how those with health and mobility needs fare in market sector, especially in the majority home ownership tenure (Easterlow *et al.* 2000). The under-representation of sick and disabled people in the home ownership sector may reflect constraints on access to the tenure. Qualitative interviews with home owners who experienced health problems raised issues around securing finance, finding a suitable property and sustaining home ownership. The researchers concluded that the sustainability of home ownership for those at the margins of the tenure needed to be seen as an emerging public health issue (Easterlow *et al.* 2000).

There is increasing recognition of (and research evidence for) the negative impact of inappropriate housing on the mental health of occupants. Many of the issues relate to needs for care and support in addition to housing, or to the experience of homelessness, as considered in the following sections.

Health, care and support within the dwelling

Appropriate housing alone is not always sufficient to meet the health and social care needs of some households. There are physical and mental health care needs associated with the key client groups for Care in the Community, and resettlement and support needs associated with other vulnerable groups. This is a key area for joint working between housing, health and social care professionals.

The policy of caring for vulnerable people in the community – as far as possible in their own homes – rather than in large de-personalised institutions has developed gradually over the last 30 years. Although social services and health authorities have been the lead agencies, housing is a key building block in making the policy work (Audit Commission 1998). The success of community care as a policy therefore lies in effectively supporting people with a range of physical and mental health needs in ordinary housing.

People are living longer and many elderly people need support to stay in their own homes. The number of older people with mental health problems is growing rapidly. The number over 65 is predicted to rise by 10 per cent in the next ten years with the greatest increase amongst the over 80s. These 'older' old will need the most help from services (Audit Commission 2000). Housing authorities are struggling to cope with demand and are constrained by the stock of social housing available. Much social housing stock is unsuitable for community care clients with frail older people or those with physical disabilities waiting up to two years for routine adaptations to property. Specialised accommodation including sheltered housing for older people is not always located where need is greatest. Not only is the delay distressing to users but additional costs are incurred through more demands on home-care and the increased risk of institutional solutions (Audit Commission 1998).

Increasing numbers of people with mental health problems are housed in the community. Research has shown that good quality, well-managed housing can be the single most important factor for

successful community care for people with mental health problems (Thompson *et al.* 1995). While specialist support can be provided by health and social services teams, feeling safe and secure
at home is fundamental to well-being. Equally, adequate housing
alone is unlikely to be sufficient to ensure those with mental health
problems live securely in the community.

A key problem lies in achieving a balance between normalisa-
tion and social isolation (Quilgars 1998). If vulnerable people
living in mainstream accommodation do not receive basic support –
with budgeting, shopping and other everyday skills that most take
for granted – they may fall into difficulty leading to a distressing
chain of events. A problem may precipitate hospitalisation,
followed by resettlement into social housing with minimal or no
support until the next crisis occurs. In effect many become
trapped in a 'revolving door' syndrome – where households lack
the skills, resources or support services to cope with independent
living, possibly resulting in tenancy difficulties, eviction and subsequent homelessness (Chartered Institute of Housing 1998). It has
been argued that support has been tied too closely to properties
(e.g. sheltered/specialist housing) rather than to the people who
live in them. Further, resources have tended to be locked into crisis management rather than prevention. Both such strategies have
led to mismatches with real need as experienced by service users.
It has been established that the greater the quantity, but especially
the better the quality of social support available to those with
mental health problems, the better their long-term health status in
the community is likely to be (Dunn 2000).

Despite widespread acceptance of the principals of care in the
community, the research literature continues to identify inadequa-
cies in practice and dissatisfaction in the lived experience of service users (Farrell *et al.* 1999). Most care groups desired choice
about where to live and access to community life, but many could
not afford to move from problem areas. Many also felt isolated and
that they were not listened to or asked for opinions. Some older
people were living in residential homes which were unsuitable
properties with too many stairs or insufficient space, but there was
little alternative choice (Farrell *et al.* 1999).

An important way forward is for the housing, health and care
professions to ensure that people with health problems and mobility needs have a fair chance of avoiding harmful environments and

of accessing homes which are enabling rather than disabling (Easterlow *et al.* 2000). Improvement lies in the building of effective partnerships across housing, health and social services to make best use of resources and to provide flexible care that meets the needs of both users and carers (Audit Commission 1998).

A number of initiatives which can help secure improved outcomes have been recommended by the Chartered Institute for Housing (CIH), the professional organisation for housing. Among those recommended are joint training and liaison meetings; agreed arrangements regarding the preparation and review of individual community care assessments and care plans; ongoing support for vulnerable individuals; and procedures to identify tenants with health problems caused or compounded by lack of support (Chartered Institute of Housing 1998). Without such safeguards, a proportion of people who could otherwise live independently with support, will run the risk of homelessness, with associated public health outcomes as discussed below.

Health and homelessness

Homelessness remains an enduring social issue in the United Kingdom. Despite the existence of legislation to protect some households in the event of homelessness, the experience remains a traumatic one for those affected (Clapham and Hutson 1999). The statutory process is complex but local housing authorities retain a duty to provide accommodation for households who are deemed unintentionally homeless and in priority need. Priority need categories include households made homeless in an emergency and those with dependent children, an expectant mother, someone over retirement age or someone deemed 'vulnerable' due to illness/disability or other limited special circumstances. Most single people of working age were excluded from the statutory provisions introduced in 1977 and they comprised the main group who experienced absolute rooflessness (also known as street homelessness or sleeping rough) in increasing numbers during the 1980s and 1990s (Burrows *et al.* 1997).

Research and policy reports have increasingly acknowledged that there are a whole host of health issues relating to homelessness. Indeed, arguably, it is homeless households who nowadays experience the most severe housing-related health issues. While family households may have priority for access to social housing, a great deal of stress is still associated with the crisis of homelessness (Chartered Institute of Housing 1998). Living in temporary accommodation and permanent relocation may involve moving to a different (probably less desirable) area, entailing changes in schooling for children and possibly changing GP registration. Children of homeless families suffer specific health risks, such as delayed social and physical development, behavioural problems and increased risk of both accidental and non-accidental injury (Chartered Institute of Housing 1998).

Homeless single people without children, often living in hostel accommodation or sleeping rough, are known to experience particularly severe health/social problems (including the re-emergence of tuberculosis) and reduced mortality (Chartered Institute of Housing 1998). Disrupted lives from early years, including a history of care, offending, poor educational attainment, unemployment and alcohol/drug abuse are all associated with the most severe experience of homelessness (Anderson *et al.* 1993; Bines 1997; Yanetta *et al.* 1999; Fitzpatrick *et al.* 2000). Research evidence has highlighted problems of access to basic health care for single homeless people. Many are not registered with a GP, due to a combination of practical problems relating to not having a fixed address, coupled with a degree of discrimination. Where homeless people do attend for treatment, there can be serious problems in tracing their medical records and ensuring appropriate follow-up treatment (Pleace *et al.* 2000). A key health issue identified by an evaluation of the Scottish initiative to tackle street homelessness was the shortage of suitable detoxification and rehabilitation facilities (and suitable move on accommodation) for homeless people with drug and alcohol dependency problems (Yanetta *et al.* 1999).

A high proportion of single homeless people report having some form of mental health problem, ranging from anxiety/depression, through substance abuse to more severe mental health issues (Bines 1997). However, research evidence to date is inconclusive as to whether mental health problems precede or follow homelessness (Craig *et al.* 1996; Watson 1999). The reality is likely to be a mixture of the two scenarios. While there is an association between the closure of long stay mental institutions and the

increase of mental health problems among the homeless population, this does not necessarily relate to inappropriate hospital discharge procedures in a straightforward way. Issues around
the breakdown of community care arrangements have been identified, but Craig and Timms (1992) also point to the closure of
large hostels which may have previously 'hidden' mental illness
issues among residents.

Young people (aged under 25 years) are over-represented
among the single homeless population in Britain and research evidence suggests their mental health and well-being suffers acutely.
Moreover, the mental health needs of young homeless people
appeared to become increasingly severe during the 1990s, placing
pressure on support agencies to tackle difficult issues which had
not previously been within their remit (Watson 1999). Young people from minority ethnic groups who become homeless may face
additional exclusion where service provision is insensitive to cultural needs or language issues, or they simply feel uncomfortable
using white-dominated services (Small and Hinton 1997). The
impact of homelessness on the physical and mental well-being of
vulnerable young people is of particular concern given that Marsh
et al. (2000) have established that the consequences of poor housing for poor health extend across the life course.

Housing, health and multiple disadvantage

A number of broad conclusions emerge from a review of research
on housing and health. First associations between housing and
health exist and the research evidence supports the argument that
good quality housing has an important role to play in achieving
good health outcomes (Wilkinson 1999). However, the evidence
from differing studies has not been entirely consistent and debates
as to why there are few proven causal relationships have hinged
around methodological constraints. Rather than pursue the difficult route of proving cause and effect further, it may be more productive to accept that associations exist and that housing clearly
plays an important role in relation to general health and well-being
(Wilkinson 1999).

More recently a stronger case has been made for a direct
causal relationship between poor housing and poor health

(Marsh *et al.* 2000). While the 1990s saw a renewed interest in understanding the relationships between housing and health, these relationships have become increasingly complex, with less of a clear technical explanatory basis (Whitehead 2000; Dunn 2000). Consequently, modern policy solutions are less obvious and more difficult to measure, than with, say, remedying dampness/unfitness or alleviating infectious diseases.

Irrespective of cause and effect, the evidence demonstrates a range of ways in which housing and health are inter-related. Yet, these two dimensions of welfare need to be seen in relation to the other components of well-being such as income, educational attainment, employment, family support and social and community networks. While it may be difficult to establish clear cause and effect in relation to housing and health, it is evident that disadvantage in one sphere of well-being is commonly associated with compound or multiple disadvantage across a range of spheres. In the United Kingdom, such links have been explicitly acknowledged by the New Labour governments elected in 1997 and 2001, and have become fundamental to the development of 'joined up' social policy under the social exclusion/inclusion agenda (Anderson 2000). The following section sets out recent housing policy developments within this broader context.

Public health under New Labour: the significance of housing

Central and local government policies and strategies are key determinants of practice and outcomes across all dimensions of welfare. This section focusses on the most recent directions for housing policy under New Labour since 1997, and considers the significance of developments in housing for public health. In doing so, it is important to note that housing is an aspect of public policy which has been particularly affected by the post-1997 implementation of devolution in the United Kingdom. The Scottish Parliament has a greater degree of autonomy than the Northern Ireland, Welsh and Greater London assemblies. In Scotland, legislative powers and full responsibility for policy in the spheres of housing and health are now devolved to the Parliament in Edinburgh. The proportional representation system for elections to the new institutions also meant that while the New Labour government in Westminster retained significant UK wide influence, some divergence in housing policy across the United Kingdom was becoming evident. New housing legislation was passed in the Parliaments in Scotland and England/Wales during 2000/2001. Both Acts contained provisions to strengthen the rights of homeless households, although English local authorities still have lesser duties than their Scottish counterparts. However, other aspects of policy and legislative change had a lot more to do with the structures and finance of rented housing rather than, for example, broad targets to improve quality or increase provision. Examples would include the introduction of a new 'Scottish Secure Tenancy' to cover both council and housing association dwellings and proposals to restructure how rents are set for council and housing association tenancies in England and Wales. For health and care workers liaising with housing agencies, it is important to be aware that the traditional system of council housing provision and needs based allocation systems is gradually being transformed into a much more diverse and complex sector (Cowan and Marsh 2001).

Arguably, the packages of measures are designed to smooth the restructuring of the social housing sector with local government focusing on a strategic enabling role and the physical provision and management of social rented housing being gradually transferred to new or existing alternative landlords. The process of stock transfer is both politically and practically contentious and is highly complex in terms of the financial arrangements for transfer. In theory, however, the new landlords should be more free than local authorities to borrow capital finance to reinvest in the fabric of the housing stock, thus contributing to improving the housing conditions and health of occupants. However, public health *per se* was not an explicit factor driving either the policy or the legislation.

Legislation is not the only policy tool available to government. Other initiatives also have a potentially significant impact upon housing, health and well-being. This is particularly the case where significant levels of government resources are committed to key political initiatives (e.g. the Rough Sleeping Initiatives in England and Scotland).

One of the earliest New Labour initiatives in 'joining up' policy and practice was the creation of the Social Exclusion Unit in 1997 (Anderson 2000). Housing related issues were prominent in the early work of the Social Exclusion Unit in England. The reduction of street homelessness was one of the government's first priorities. A detailed review process acknowledged the need for a coordinated approach to the problem which took account of the health care and support needs of homeless people, as well as their housing needs. As indicated in the research evidence described above, it was recognised that housing agencies alone could not solve street homelessness, and that health and social work agencies needed to acknowledge their potential role.

While a Rough Sleepers Initiative (RSI) had been in place since 1991, a key development from the 1998 review was the subsequent setting up of another cross-departmental unit – the Rough Sleepers Unit – specifically to oversee implementation of a coordinated strategy. A homelessness coordinator (or 'tsar') was appointed to steer through the multidimensional strategy, ensuring collaboration between all the relevant government and non-government agencies. In Scotland, an evaluation of the first phase of the Scottish RSI identified that the initiative had been largely housing led and there was a need for more equal input from health and social work agencies (Yanetta *et al.* 1999). As part of fine-tuning of the second phase of the initiative, the post of Health and Homelessness Coordinator was created in an attempt to improve collaboration across services.

Another key strand to New Labour's joined up housing strategy has been the development of a National Strategy for Neighbourhood renewal. A lengthy process of review of policy and practice culminated in the publication of the final strategy document in January 2001 (Social Exclusion Unit 2001) and the setting up of a Neighbourhood Renewal Unit to deliver the strategy. The thrust of this would be towards managing communities, rather than housing, again, recognising the impact of multiple deprivation, its geographical concentration in certain areas and the need for broad-ranging solutions to tackle deprivation across a range of social indicators.

The importance of the joined up approach is equally evident from New Labour's health policy statements, which have increasingly accepted that poor health is closely linked to poverty, unemployment, bad housing, poor education and a poor quality environment (Easterlow *et al.* 2000). For example, in Scotland, New Labour explicitly acknowledged that improved housing offers the prospect of better mental health, less sickness linked to damp and cold, and fewer accidents (Scottish Office 1999). Since the Acheson Report (1998) highlighted housing and environment as key areas for future policy development if health inequalities were to be reduced, the link between housing and health has continued to move up the political agenda (Marsh *et al.* 2000). For example, the White Paper, *Saving Lives – Our Healthier Nation* (Department of Health 1999) also recognised housing as one of the key environmental factors which affect health, and housing features prominently in high profile health initiatives such as Health Action Zones.

With the publication of the White Papers, *The New NHS – Modern and Dependable* (Department of Health 1997) and *Saving Lives*, the Government signalled a determination to tackle the root causes of ill-health and placed the reduction of health inequalities at the centre of health policy. With this has come a greater acknowledgement of the wider social, economic and environmental causes of ill-health (Molyneux 2000). The White Papers set frameworks for improving the delivery of health services and health improvements. These frameworks such as Health Improvement Programmes (HIP), Health Action Zones (HAZ), and Healthy Living Centres seek to create new partnerships to improve health and health care and give new energy to local activity that tackles the causes of poor health such as education, employment, housing and community safety. Meanwhile, services such as NHS Direct and the introduction of Primary Care Groups (PCGs) and Primary Care Trusts (PCTs) signal an intention to radically alter the perception of health services at a community level. The increasing profile of housing issues in HIP and HAZ plans demonstrates that the new frameworks are already delivering a higher profile for wider environmental and public health issues in multi-agency approaches to health promotion and health care.

The period from May 1997 to the end of 2001 can be characterised as one of review and policy development, with the beginnings of implementation of New Labour's joined up strategies. Clearly the recognition of policy linkages and structures for collaborative working pre-date the New Labour government, but the post-1997 era has been one in which 'joined up' thinking and working has been given much higher priority than previously. This approach presents new challenges for housing and public health professionals in delivering quality services both within and across traditional professional boundaries. A key task for new research on housing and public health will be to assess the outcomes and effectiveness of the approaches outlined. The final section gives an initial assessment of changing practice.

Housing and health: developments in practice

The CIH publishes guidance on good practice in housing, including specific recommendations on housing/homelessness and health (Chartered Institute of Housing 1998). While such guidance does draw on published research, it also emerges from agreed consensus among practitioners as to what, precisely constitutes good practice. Recommendations will be influenced by contemporary policy developments as well as examples from 'lead' organisations. Such guidance, whilst acknowledged by the profession, must be treated with some caution as examples cited have not necessarily been the subject of rigorous independent evaluation. Guidance as recommended by the professional body is advisory and not mandatory for public or voluntary sector housing agencies. Nevertheless, such guidance does give a helpful indication of the contemporary state of the art in housing practice relating to health and well-being. Government departments may also produce guidance to support new policy initiatives or legislative changes.

Health and housing good practice

First and foremost, there is an expectation that health and housing agencies will examine the links across their work and develop appropriate strategies for collaborative working. The CIH advocates multi-agency working and the breaking down of professional barriers across housing, health, social services and other relevant agencies. The requirement is to work in partnership towards common objectives. Key areas for joint initiatives include health care for homeless people, medical assessment for rehousing in the social sector, hospital discharge procedures and appropriate housing and support for people with disabilities and mental health problems. The CIH publishes detailed working guidance for agencies and examples of existing inter-agency projects (Chartered Institute of Housing 1998).

It is recommended that health objectives are integrated into the housing strategies and programmes set by local authorities and other housing agencies. Potential health outcomes should be considered when deciding on investment priorities for housing. Strategies to improve housing conditions, including regeneration, affordable warmth and home safety should lead to improved health outcomes over the long term. Other key steps which housing agencies can take to improve the health of local people include helping to tackle crime (e.g. installing closed circuit television (CCTV)) and providing mediation services to resolve neighbour disputes (assisting mental health). Community regeneration, stock renovation and environmental initiatives also offer opportunities to secure better living conditions, provide local employment and achieve public health gains. It is also recommended that both landlords and tenants are involved in identifying community health initiatives. The idea of empowering residents is considered important to increasing self-esteem, building up community confidence and thereby contributing to enhanced well-being.

Health and homelessness good practice

It is strongly recommended, by the CIH, that local authorities should aim to rehouse homeless households directly into 'good quality permanent stock' when possible, whilst minimising the use of temporary accommodation. It is also acknowledged that housing agencies should avoid placing vulnerable people in unsupported temporary accommodation. Where temporary accommodation is used, it should be of good quality standards relating to health, safety, space, warmth and management, with systems to inspect and monitor conditions. Detailed guidance is also provided in relation to medical priorities for rehousing within the social rented sector (Chartered Institute of Housing 1998).

The CIH also recommends ongoing liaison with health and welfare agencies in relation to homeless households. This would include negotiating appropriate support and care packages and appropriate access to day centres, play groups and so on. Housing agencies are also encouraged to provide homeless households with information and advice on access to primary and emergency health services, including registering with a GP.

A key issue for debate is the appropriateness of the provision of health services specifically for homeless people. While homeless people remain excluded from mainstream services, however, there is likely to remain a need for specialist provision and outreach staff. Health services which can be delivered direct to homeless people (and tailored to meet their needs) include specialist GP surgeries along with podiatry, dental and Community Psychiatric Nurse services.

The extent to which the above good practice recommendations are put into effective practice is likely to be variable. The pressures on local housing systems can vary significantly in different parts of the United Kingdom as can the effectiveness with which housing and health agencies work together. Overall, research evidence to date would suggest that while significant progress has been made in delivering more coherent, joined up services, too many vulnerable clients are still failed through lack of coordination and sheer lack of resources.

Conclusion

This chapter has focused on the links between housing and health and the potential for joint working to improve public health outcomes. However, the degree of overlap does need to be kept in perspective. As Allen (2001) has argued, there are people who live in poor housing who do not become ill and people who live in high quality housing who experience severe health problems. The relationships are not simplistic and joint working will not be appropriate in every circumstance. Nevertheless, the contemporary themes of coordination and collaboration in order to tackle multiple disadvantage seem well embedded in the policy framework at the beginning of the twenty-first century. While the theories, policies and strategies seem well established, implementation through practical interventions remains at a relatively early stage. A key challenge for the immediate future is to monitor the effectiveness of joined up working and to identify outcomes for housing, public health and quality of life in a meaningful way. There remains a need for a comprehensive medium-long term assessment of whether the United Kingdom has become a better housed and healthier nation under New Labour.

References

Acheson Report (1998) *Independent inquiry into inequalities in health.* Stationery Office, London.

Allen C (2001) On the 'physiological dope' problematic in housing and illness research: towards a critical realism of home and health. *Housing, Theory and Society* 17(2): 49–67.

Allen T (2000) Housing renewal – doesn't it make you sick? *Housing Studies* 15(3): 443–60.

Anderson I (1993) Housing policy and street homelessness in Britain. *Housing Studies* 8(1): 17–28.

Anderson I (1994) Access to housing for low income single people. Centre for Housing Policy, University of York.

Anderson I (2000) 'Social exclusion: the changing debate' in Anderson I and Sim D (eds) *Housing and Social Exclusion: Context and Challenges.* Chartered Institute of Housing and Housing Studies Association, Coventry, chapter 2, pp 6–21.

Anderson I and Sim D (eds) (2000) *Housing and Social Exclusion: Context and Challenges.* Chartered Institute of Housing and Housing Studies Association, Coventry.

Anderson I, Kemp P and Quilgars D (1993) *Single Homeless People.* HMSO, London.

Audit Commission (1998) *Home Alone: The Role of Housing in Community Care.* Audit Commission, London.

Audit Commission (2000) *Forget Me Not: Mental Health Services for Older People.* Audit Commission, Abingdon.

Bines W (1997) 'The health of single homeless people' in Burrows R, Pleace N and Quilgars D (eds) *Homelessness and Social Policy.* Routledge, London, chapter 9, pp 132–49.

Burrows R, Pleace N and Quilgars D (eds) (1997) *Homelessness and Social Policy.* Routledge, London.

Chartered Institute of Housing (1998) *Good Practice Briefing: Housing and Health.* Chartered Institute of Housing, Coventry.

Clapham D and Hutson S (eds) (1999) *Homelessness: Public Policies and Private Troubles.* Cassals, London.

Cooper C and Hawtin M (eds) (1998) *Resident Involvement and Community Action: Theory to Practice.* Chartered Institute of Housing, Coventry.

Cowan D and Marsh A (eds) (2001) *Two Steps Forward: Housing Policy into the New Millennium.* The Policy Press, Bristol.

Craig T, Hodson S, Woodward S and Richardson S (1996) *Off to a Bad Start: A Longitudinal Study of Homeless Young People in London.* The Mental Health Foundation, London.

Craig T and Timms P (1992) Out of the wars and onto the streets? Deinstitutionalisation and homelessness in Britain. *UK J Ment Health* **1**(3): 265–75.

Department of Health (1997) *The New NHS: Modern and Dependable.* White Paper. Cmnd 3807. The Stationary Office, London.

Department of Health (1999) *Saving Lives: Our Healthier Nation.* White Paper. Cmnd 4386. The Stationery Office, London.

Dunn J (2000) Housing and health inequalities: review and prospects for research. *Housing Studies* **15**(3): 341–66.

Easterlow D, Smith SJ and Mallinson S (2000) Housing for health: the role for owner occupation. *Housing Studies* **15**(3): 367–86.

Ellaway A, Fairley A and Macintyre S (1999) *Housing Improvement and Health Improvement in Inverclyde.* A report commissioned by the Inverclyde Regeneration Partnership.

Farrell C, Robinson J and Fletcher P (1999) *A New Era for Community Care? What People Want from Health, Housing and Social Care Services.* King's Fund, London.

Fitzpatrick S, Kemp P and Klinker S (2000) *Single Homelessness: An Overview of Research in Britain.* Policy Press, Bristol.

Ford J (1993) Mortgage possession. *Housing Studies* **8**(4): 227–40.

Greve J and Currie E (1990) *Homelessness in Britain.* Joseph Rowntree Foundation, York.

Guardian (2000) A healthy outlook. *Society.* 11 October, p 2.

Kearns A, Hiscock R, Ellaway A and Macintyre S (2000) 'Beyond four walls'. The psycho-social benefits of home: evidence from West Central Scotland. *Housing Studies* **15**(3): 387–410.

Kemp P (1999) 'Housing Policy under New Labour, Chapter' in Powell M (ed.) *New Labour, New Welfare State: The 'Third Way' in British Social Policy.* The Policy Press, Bristol.

Lowe S (2000) 'Housing abandonment' in Anderson I and Sim D (eds) *Social Exclusion and Housing: Context and Challenges.* Chartered Institute of Housing, Coventry, chapter 12, pp 177–90.

Malpass P and Murie A (1999) *Housing Policy and Practice.* 5th edn. Macmillan, London.

Marsh A, Gordon D, Heslop P and Pantazis C (2000) Housing deprivation and health: a longitudinal analysis. *Housing Studies* **15**(3): 411–28.

Molyneux P (2000) *Forging the Link: Health and Housing in the West Midlands.* National Housing Federation, Birmingham.

Mullen T (2001) 'Stock transfer' in Cowan D and Marsh A (eds) *Two Steps Forward: Housing Policy into the New Millennium.* The Policy Press, Bristol, chapter 3, pp 47–67.

Murie A and Nevin B (2001) 'New Labour transfers' in Cowan D and Marsh A (eds) *Two Steps Forward: Housing Policy into the New Millennium.* The Policy Press, Bristol, chapter 2, pp 29–45.

Nettleton S and Burrows R (2000) When a capital investment becomes an emotional loss: the health consequences of the experience of mortgage possession in England. *Housing Studies* 15(3): 463–79.

O'Carroll A (1996) 'Historical perspectives on tenure development in urban Scotland' in Currie H and Murie A (eds) *Housing in Scotland.* Chartered Institute of Housing, Coventry, chapter 2, pp 16–30.

Oldman C and Beresford B (2000) Home, sick home: using the housing experiences of disabled children to suggest a new theoretical framework. *Housing Studies* 15(3): 429–42.

Pleace N, Jones A and England J (2000) *Access to General Practice for People Sleeping Rough.* Centre for Housing Policy/Department of Health, York.

Quilgars D (1998) *A Life in the Community. Home-Link: Supporting people with mental health problems in ordinary housing.* The Policy Press, Bristol.

Revell K and Leather P (2000) *The State of UK Housing: A Factfile on Housing Conditions and Housing Renewal Policies in the UK.* 2nd edn. The Policy Press, Bristol.

Scottish Office (1999) *Towards a Healthier Scotland: A White Paper on Health.* The Stationary Office, Edinburgh.

Social Exclusion Unit (2001) *A New Commitment to Neighbourhood Renewal: National Strategy Action Plan.* The Stationary Office, London.

Small C and Hinton T (1997) *Reaching Out: A Study of Black and Minority Ethnic Single Homelessness and Access to Primary Health Care.* Health Action for Homeless People, London.

Smith SJ, Alexander A and Easterlow D (1998) Rehousing as a health intervention: miracle or mirage. *Health and Place* 3: 203–16.

Thompson K, Phelan M, Strathdee G and Shires D (1995) *Mental Health Care: A Guide for Housing Workers.* The Mental Health Foundation, London.

Universities of Sussex and Westminster (1996) *The Real Cost of Poor Homes.* Royal Institute for Chartered Surveyors, London.

Watson L (1999) *Not Mad, Bad or Young Enough: Helping Young Homeless People with Mental Health Problems.* The Policy Press, Bristol.

Whitehead C (2000) Editorial (Special issue on housing and health). *Housing Studies* 15(3): 339–40.

Wilcox S (2000) *Housing Finance Review 2000/2001.* Chartered Institute of Housing, Coventry. Council of Mortgage Lenders, London. Joseph Rowntree Foundation, York.

Wilkinson D (1999) *Poor Housing and Ill Health: A Summary of Research Evidence.* Scottish Office Central Research Unit, Edinburgh.

Yanetta A, Third H and Anderson I (1999) *National Monitoring and Interim Evaluation of the Rough Sleeping Initiative in Scotland.* Scottish Executive Central Research Unit, Edinburgh.

8

Environmental Health

John Wildsmith, Paul Belcher,
Gary Mumford and Colin Powell

Introduction

The environmental health profession has a long history, from the formation of the local government system in the United Kingdom. Its development has in many instances been in response to factors which have a demonstrable impact upon the health of communities. The discipline of environmental health covers a broad range of specialist fields including food safety, housing, occupational health and safety, and pollution control. Additionally, the means by which these functions are undertaken are multi-faceted, including the application of skills in monitoring, inspection, enforcement education and advising. In order to achieve success in such a range of activities, the environmental health practitioner has had to develop a broad range of skills and competencies, which are focussed upon providing a public health protection service to the public at large.

This chapter therefore highlights a number of these key skills and how they may be utilised by practitioners. It also seeks to comment on the influences that have shaped the nature of the environmental health service.

Evidence of current government thinking, such as the views expressed in Saving Lives – Our Healthier Nation (HMSO 1999a), suggests that delivery of public health services is in transition. It is therefore timely that there is an evaluation of the contribution and working methods of the environmental health profession and their role within the field of public health. This evaluation should involve a review of the use of evidence-based approaches to intervention, interfacing with local communities and the process of risk assessment. An important aspect of such times of transition is that they present opportunities to re-evaluate traditional models of service delivery, in order to ensure that they are providing the expected or predicted outputs to the correct target group.

The current system for the delivery of the environmental health service in the United Kingdom stems from the reorganisation of local government in 1974. Responsibilities and functions formerly undertaken by public health departments were firmly embedded in the district-level local authorities. In this sense the environmental health practitioner might be considered to represent a professional, technical function, which has evolved from the earliest manifestations of the local government structure.

During this reorganisation, other public health functions, such as that of the Medical Officer of Health, were removed from the local government framework and transferred to new National Health Service structures. Since that time there has been an ongoing debate concerning the appropriateness of such a divide in what many consider should be a holistic function and recent government publications (HMSO 1999a, 2000a) and those of bodies such as the King's Fund (Gowman and Coote 2000) and Chartered Institute of Environmental Health (CIEH 1997) have questioned such a division of roles.

Many commentators in the United Kingdom have called for greater integration of the current public health service and the environmental health service. In addition, organisations such as the World Health Organisation have stated that partnerships should be developed with sectors beyond those traditionally designated as having responsibility for the protection and enhancement of public health. This approach can be considered at both the macro (national and international level) and the micro (community/ local) level. Such services are normally regarded as being most effectively delivered at a community level involving close collaboration between the key actors, and this requires a coordinated, strategic approach to the delivery of a new form of public health, which can demonstrate effective communication between all stakeholders.

At the heart of the debate is the apparent conflict between those who espouse the medical model of health and those who prefer to advocate a social view of health. Many critics of Our Healthier Nation argue that the public health strategy advocated in this document, is firmly located within a medical model. The emphasis on lifestyle issues and matters closely linked to the performance of acute health services, coupled with the apparent absence of any reference to wider factors such as the environment, would tend to support this view, and possibly highlights the tension between the various professional groups involved.

It is perhaps worthy of consideration that any such tensions can lead to differences in opinion of the value of the environmental health function. These tensions which are quite common between professional groups which perceive themselves to be in competition, will undoubtedly consume significant time and energy from all parties, and whatever the outcome, it is unlikely that the individuals or communities for whom the services exist, will benefit.

Agendas for Change

One of the most significant developments of the late twentieth century was the establishment of a Commission on Environmental Health in 1996, by the Chartered Institute of Environmental Health, created with support from the Royal Environmental Health Institute of Scotland, the City of Edinburgh Council and Oxford City Council.

The Commission essentially expressed the view that 'health and the environment have always been intimately related' (CIEH 1997). This echoes the observation that whilst poor environments are well understood to be a cause of ill-health, high quality environments can contribute directly to improvement and maintenance of a better quality of life, and well-being.

This view concerning the impact of environmental factors on the public health has developed from the basic sanitary reforms of the nineteenth century, which attempted to bring (amongst other things) satisfactory housing accommodation with clean drinking water supplies as well as suitable and sufficient sewage handling systems and adequate waste collection and disposal facilities to the populace. In fact, it can be argued that many of the original problems concerning the health of the population caused by poor housing and associated services are still with us today. For example, regular house condition surveys, undertaken by the government, indicate that a significant proportion of the nation's housing stock, is either in an unsatisfactory state of repair or even unfit for human habitation. Whilst area renewal and revitalising policies have come and gone, involving significant cost to the government purse by way of grants, there are still areas in many parts of the country, both urban and rural, where large numbers of properties are in an extremely poor condition, and the health of the occupants is clearly at risk.

Similarly, whilst drinking water quality has undoubtedly improved, concerns relating to levels of pesticides and occasional but noteworthy outbreaks of Cryptosporidiosis demonstrate that all is far from ideal in terms of current risks to public health from these environmental factors. Blocked and defective drains still constitute a significant level of complaint for local authorities and the taking of enforcement action is still an important part of the daily work of many environmental health practitioners.

However, in addition to what may be considered to be the more traditional environmental health problems, there are new and perhaps more complex issues which require a broader range of expertise to solve. Perhaps at this point it would be helpful to consider the model of an orchestra, to reflect the expertise required. Here, each of the main sections of the orchestra has their individual roles to play, defined by the limits of the score. No instrument is allowed to start using the music intended for another section. However, each section playing in its own time will not deliver the intended outcome. Indeed it is only when there is a coordinated, precise unification of sections that the overall impression intended by the composer can be realised. Of course, one extremely important factor is the control and coordination imposed by a conductor, who achieves the end result. To conclude the analogy, there must also be an audience to receive the end result and who, if suitably impressed, will applaud the players. It is possible to make a strong case that the environmental health practitioner, with a range of scientific, technical, legal and social skills is in a strong position to participate in this process in order to deliver an effective public health service to the community.

The Commission on Environmental Health, in its introductory remarks, commented on the view that the linkage between health and environment may have tended to drift apart, 'both conceptually and in our institutions'. They pursue this aspect of the problem by commenting that 'health policy, resources and institutions have concentrated mainly on care and treatment of the unhealthy, with prevention taking too much of a second place' (CIEH 1997).

To be able to understand the current position, we must examine the interface between health policy and environmental policy in the United Kingdom. We also need to examine the level of integration of the various actors, in order to consider the consequences for public health in the future, and in particular, to consider the sustainability of the environmental health system.

'Agendas for Change' considered that there should be a clear and consistent vision of environmental health if the strategic planning and management of a service to the public is to be provided. The document does pose a number of questions, which really need to be addressed if the value of an environmental health service is to be justified. Drawing on a food-based analogy, the question is put as to whether the familiar model of environmental health, established in the days of Victorian Britain, is 'now well past its use-by date'.

This is a very pertinent question, which needs to be addressed by professional bodies and political decision-takers alike. Agendas for Change also considered a broad view of environmental health in its vision for the year 2020, and in summary, reflects the belief that the best organisational model for the delivery of good environmental health services is a local one. The Commission also considered that any new organisational structures must be 'flexible, inclusive and task-orientated'. It is made clear that these structures must include inputs from local communities and locally based professionals, without defining the balance, but they neatly state that 'the professionals will be on tap rather than on top'. Clearly this is attesting that the current systems for delivery of an environmental health service are easily dominated by professionals with their own agenda which may or may not address the needs of the client groups.

Another important aspect of Agendas for Change is the consideration of the training of environmental health practitioners. At present this training is controlled by the core curricula developed by the various professional bodies. Universities and colleges are required to adhere to this as a basis for their teaching. In the case of environmental health officers, academic theory is supplemented by practical training for one year. This is assessed by the completion of a training logbook and a series of professional interviews. Once a trainee has successfully completed the academic and practical training periods, they may become registered by the professional body and they are then able to fully enter professional practice.

A tension can arise, however, when emphasis is placed on the acquisition of measurable technical competence. Environmental health is not only about the practical application of technical and scientific knowledge within the community. Environmental health practitioners need more than technical competence if they are to win the confidence of members of the public. There is a need for what the authors of Agendas for Change refer to as 'social skills' (CIEH 1997). Whilst the Chartered Institute of Environmental Health has an element within its logbook on 'dealing with difficult situations' there is a need for more emphasis to be placed on developing mechanisms to enable those wishing to enter this profession the opportunity to acquire these 'social skills'. These mechanisms should not only be applied to those entering the profession; there is a need for ensuring that all environmental health practitioners are assessed for their competence in this area with the use of Continuing Professional Development.

What must be addressed in the future therefore is the development of mechanisms that will ensure that environmental health practitioners are trained to work in a way that both empowers people, and promotes community development. The Commission for Environmental Health suggested that environmental health practitioners must not be trained and appointed 'merely to direct and instruct'. In fact, it is suggested that a new role is defined for environmental health practitioners in which 'they will link up organisations that have previously worked in isolation and they will be a major ingredient in the delivery of an integrated and multidisciplinary programme'. Perhaps the time has come for an independent training needs analysis to be undertaken of all professionals who contribute to public health, in whatever capacity, in order to integrate at least certain aspects of their training so that common ground can be established in relevant areas of their work.

Due to these comments as part of a vision for the future, it can be concluded that the contribution made to the protection and enhancement of public health by the environmental health service is correctly delivered at local level, but the function itself needs to be refreshed and taken back to its roots by a stronger involvement with all the stakeholders within local communities. If this action is not taken, then perhaps decision-takers might conclude that the 'use by date' has indeed been passed, and essential environmental health functions taken up by other agencies.

Whilst Agendas for Change presents a generally very positive vision for the future of environmental health as a key component of a new public health service there have been many alternative views proffered. McArthur (2001), for example, has argued that Agendas for Change was written at a time when 'things could only get better'. Therefore, whilst the themes developed in this document may still be valid, he is convinced that recent trends in government policy and local authority practice, do not necessarily make the best use of environmental health professionals, nor do they necessarily make the greatest impact on the public's health. He expresses a view, endorsed by the authors, that 'the environmental health service within local government, has continued to be pushed to the margins of mainstream public health work, through an increasing centralisation of the direction and management of service delivery' (McArthur 2001). This can be illustrated, as we shall see below, by the increased control over food safety, and more importantly the activities of local authorities, by the Food Standards Agency (FSA). Whilst no one might argue that the FSA initiatives are appropriate, one has to question how such centralised control can co-exist with the needs of local authority enforcement officers meeting the needs of local communities, and the wishes of locally elected representatives. This tension between centre and periphery can also be seen as we now move to discuss recent government initiatives in the field of public health.

Current government developments

At the same time as the production of Agendas for Change, the new Labour government started to develop its thinking on public health (HMSO 1999a). Whilst recognising the need to integrate central government and local government work to improve public health, the policies proposed for both intervention and training, focussed heavily on activities located within the National Health Service. However, this action plan did recognise the potency of social, economic and environmental factors in determining health outcomes, subsequent policy statements and resource allocation have focussed primarily on those activities associated with the medical treatment of ill-health and disease.

In contrast to this approach adopted by the Department of Health, the (then) Welsh Office in 1998, published its consultation document 'Better Health, Better Wales' (Welsh Office 1998). This set out a series of policy aims for achieving sustainable health and well-being in Wales through collaborative action. The Welsh Office recognised that most of the causes of ill-health lie outside the National Health Service, and advocated a new approach, focussing on sustainable communities and improved environment, coupled with the development of healthy lifestyles. The role of local authorities acting corporately and engaging local communities was emphasised. These local authorities were to lead newly constituted Health Alliances, which would aim to deliver sustainable local health gains. To achieve these goals however, there is a need to establish multi-dimensional means of communication, which account for local community perspectives and priorities.

It should also be noted however, that in order to effect change, there is a need to work collaboratively. However, in many cases barriers to this exist. One example of such a barrier is seen in the work commissioned by the Going for Green project funded by the Department of Environment (Centre for Environmental Sciences 1999) which highlighted that often, issues of concern identified by local communities are at variance with the intervention priorities of both those framing national policy and local service providers. In this project, when local communities were consulted in relation to their environmental concerns, they overwhelmingly reported that 'crime' and 'dog-fouling' were at the top of their agenda. This contrasted with the national focus of the project where key issues were seen to be cutting down waste, travelling sensibly, looking after the local environment, preventing pollution and saving energy and natural resources. Clearly there is a significant difference in the initial expectations of the two main groups in this particular case. Thus, when the professional groups evaluate the outcomes against the initial targets, as part of their formal research, they will tend to assume that the results are unsatisfactory. Equally, the local community will be disappointed that the published measures which reflect their own input to the process may not even address their primary concerns. This is borne out by other research (Burningham and Thrush 2001). Such studies stress the essential collaborative nature of data gathering from communities so that any expectations can be satisfied by the research methodologies employed.

The above example also highlights that, fundamental to the establishment and maintenance of effective collaborative partnerships is trust. Indicators in the Going for Green research also demonstrated that respondents had limited confidence in the ability of the local authority to listen to their concerns and to deliver appropriate local services. The issue of trust, with particular reference to the environmental health function, is considered later in this chapter.

In view of the above evidence, we must therefore consider in particular, the role of environmental health practitioners who undertake a key role in the protection of public health within local communities. Their training requires that environmental health practitioners are competent risk assessors and effective risk communicators across a wide variety of technical fields and this enables them to fulfil their overall role as risk regulators, whilst at the same time drawing together the interests of the various stakeholders in the local community. This broad training model supports the utilisation of their skills in the identification of relevant issues and the development of solutions that are relevant and acceptable to those bearing the burden of the risk.

Risk perception and communication

Communication and information provision have become increasingly important components of the relationship between private sector management, government institutions and the general public (Slovic 1987; Groth 1991). A body of knowledge has therefore been created over the past decade, which helps environmental health practitioners to understand how the public perceives risk, how the media translates this information, and how government, industry and other organisations can better relate to risk information over a wide range of disciplines (Renn and Levine 1991; Kasperson *et al.* 1988). This approach to communicating technological risk has been successfully applied in a number of sectors, especially in the chemical industry (Covello *et al.* 1988). This is reinforced by the requirements of the Control of Major Accident Hazards Regulations 1999 (COMAH). These regulations require certain industries to make available to the general public details of actual risks associated with the operation of their business. In a similar way, the development of the Integrated Pollution Prevention and Control (IPPC) regime in England and Wales has boosted the power of public inquiries. In addition, the new regime has opened out the planning process, expanded on the number of statutory consultees and improved the flow of information, particularly to the general public. The Environment Agency has utilised this general move to openness by encouraging members of the public to interrogate the Agency's website for details of local environmental risks. Environmental health practitioners must be aware, therefore, that there is a general recognition that decision-making in democratic societies is becoming more public and is increasingly driven by non-experts. Thus, there is a need for a risk communication framework, which acknowledges this transition.

Environmental health practitioners are becoming increasingly involved in issues where potential wide-scale risks to public health and safety are reflected in their developing role in the preparation of off-site emergency plans under the COMAH Regulations 1999 (HMSO 1999b). Such a function demonstrates the need for collaboration in a multi-disciplinary decision-making process whereby on-site and off-site emergency plans must be properly integrated, including the involvement of members of the at-risk communities in the development of documentation and procedures in a transparent, multi-directional process. Even further, to be effective, off-site emergency plans are required to be periodically rehearsed, to ensure that they are effective. Such public rehearsals may serve to illustrate limitations of decision-taking and professional judgement.

In the authors' own experience, the fear of an accidental release from a chemical store in a community, can be extremely high. The existence of central government guidance, such as PPG23 (DoE 1994) which requires that local planning authorities and their advisors should not second guess the regulators whose function it is to ensure that appropriate legal standards are being implemented, is not realistic or helpful. This is an example of outmoded thinking, which does not have a place in modern environmental health practice.

This raises an important ethical role for local government concerning the release of information gained as a result of their regulatory activities. It can be argued that in areas of potentially high consequence risk, but low probability environmental health practitioners and government might adopt a cautious approach to the release of information, so as not to create alarmist warnings of impending catastrophe. However, there are considerable problems associated with the suppression of information, especially when the potential impacts of the activity can be considerable. Indeed, in such cases, the public is likely to demand full disclosure from public servants. The BSE crisis in the United Kingdom serves to illustrate the nature of this dilemma. Here was a case of considerable scientific uncertainty, in which there was no clear burden of proof on the part of the various players in the debate. As a consequence, the government appeared to have taken a 'wait and see' approach to the problem (Phillips Report 2000).

The Royal Society (1992) highlighted that public input is vital in effective risk communication. Obtaining meaningful public input begins with the recognition that public perceptions of risk are often quite divergent from that of the scientific or expert community. 'Public reactions to risk sometimes seem bizarre, at least when compared with scientific estimates ... however, such reactions are not totally unpredictable, or even necessarily unreasonable' (DoH 1997).

The way in which people react has been the basis of much risk perception research and especially looking at those factors that shape an individual's response. These 'fright' or 'dread' factors are those, which tend to make public health risks more worrying or less acceptable (DoH 1997). It must be considered essential for all environmental health managers and practitioners to be aware of such factors and the implications for the local population when public health policies are declared or operational environmental health decisions are made.

It appears to be clear that, in order to create a sustainable system for the protection of public health it is essential to consider the range of methodologies available, the possible 'partners' who should be involved in strategy development and delivery, and the range of settings and sectors within which efforts are best targeted.

As mentioned earlier, environmental health practitioners are required to demonstrate a wide range of skills to bring about improvements to public health. The following sections contain examples of the practical aspects of the environmental health service.

Food safety

To ensure the delivery of an appropriate food safety system, we need to consider a series of elements including, environmental control (physical), education (management and food handlers and public), domestic (public), producers (hygiene and labelling) and vendors.

Overall there has to be a system of public protection, which means that the adoption of a system for visiting the target premises based upon some scale for the rating of risks posed. A question must be asked of the law enforcement system, that is, should there be a body of public officials with the skill to advise, educate and where necessary, enforce the relevant legislation to ensure that the targets are met? The question for the enforcers is what is the role; inspection or auditing of premises? Also, who actually sets the targets?

Recent developments of legislation, guidance and the development of management systems controlled by published standards or codes of practice, such as Hazard Analysis and Critical Control Points (HACCP), provide an effective framework for an audit process whereby enforcers might become the third party auditors. HACCP provides an internationally recognised framework to identify food safety hazards and the stages in the production of food which are critical to their control, in order to achieve acceptable levels of protection for the consumer.

One important aspect of food safety is related to the incidence of food-borne disease which is an issue which environmental health practitioners have been involved with for many years. The target may well be to reduce the reported incidence of food poisoning by a set amount compared to current figures. The question must be put – can reported food poisoning levels be reduced by more visits to food premises?

In recent times duties have been placed on operators of certain food businesses, to demonstrate competence in food safety. The implementation of HACCP is seen by the FSA as central to improvements being made. In fact the FSA has set itself a Service Delivery Agreement target in November 2001 for 30 per cent of food businesses to be operating documented HACCP-based control systems by April 2004 (FSA 2001). This target is set to complement wider action, which includes input by environmental health practitioners at local authority level, to reduce food-borne disease by 20 per cent by April 2006.

A local authority survey recently estimated that only 20 per cent of restaurants and other catering premises have a documented HACCP in place and 35 per cent of food premises are estimated to have no formal food safety management system in place (FSA 2001).

Scientific, risk-based approaches to delivering food safety will not, however, be sufficient on their own. A broader view should be encouraged, for instance, the labelling of foodstuffs, so that vendors and the public know exactly how to store, prepare and use high-risk food. Education is an important component of the overall need to improve food safety and there are already some environmental health practitioners who collaborate with local schools to inform the debate in the classroom. However, a greater need is to influence curriculum development as a knowledge of food safety and how to prevent illness must be seen as an important factor in the development of any society.

Again, community expectations must be addressed and the media must be used to communicate good practice. For example, the Chartered Institute of Environmental Health has sponsored a Curry Chef of the Year competition as part of their annual professional gathering. This sends out positive signals to the community.

The environmental health service makes a key contribution to the investigation of outbreaks of food-borne disease in the community. Participation involves the taking of samples for analysis, the taking of relevant statements, the inspection of premises and where appropriate, the instigation of legal proceedings. Such activities provide an essential tool for the reduction of food-borne disease in the community.

Finally, the FSA is responsible for setting and monitoring standards and auditing local authority food safety enforcement. As a part of this function, the FSA has recently issued guidance on how local authorities are expected to undertake their duties and as part of this, they are required to produce an annual Food Safety Service Plan which must be reviewed annually. The FSA guidance stresses that local authorities should adopt such plans which reflect a balance of techniques and approaches that ensure the well-being of the public, by targeting resources towards those premises which pose the greatest risk.

Initiatives such as this will require a significant level of policing. However, the success of the concept will be measured against changes in food safety statistics. When linked to measures of community involvement and planning as well as Best Value, an interesting overall picture should be revealed, driven by the actions of the environmental health practitioners.

The BSE debate

In the field of public health, the role of the environmental health practitioner is not always clearly defined. This lack of definition may be detected by both practitioners and also the other stakeholders. An example of this lack of clear definition is the debate over BSE. Mature reflection on the events surrounding this issue may lead many to feel that the environmental health practitioners' role was marginalised in a debate dominated by government officials and independent scientists.

Ministers attempted to reassure the beef-eating public that the risks from consuming beef (and by implication, beef products) were negligible. Statements were made by senior politicians and civil servants to the effect that there was no need to be worried about BSE in the United Kingdom. A series of reassurances were given by senior government figures after a dairy farmer died of Creutzfeldt Jakob Disease in 1993, and again, as late as 1995, John Major, the then Prime Minister, sought to reassure the nation by stating that he had been advised that beef was a safe and wholesome product (Phillips Report 2000). Yet, these reassurances were made against the conflicting views expressed by certain independent scientists, concerning the extent of the risks associated with the BSE contamination (Phillips Report 2000). The rigour with which policy measures were implemented for the protection of human health was affected by the belief of many prior to early 1996, that BSE was not a potential threat to human life (Smith and McCloskey 1998).

The Phillips report recognised that the government did not lie to the public about BSE. They believed that the risks posed by BSE to humans were remote and consequently, was preoccupied with preventing an alarmist over-reaction to BSE. It is now clear that this campaign of reassurance was a mistake. When on 20 March 1996 the government announced that BSE had probably been transmitted to humans, the public felt that they had been betrayed. Confidence in government pronouncements about risk was a further casualty of BSE (Phillips Report 2000).

The BSE crisis provides an ideal example of the need for accurate risk communication in the public sector; it also provides an example of the effects of poor risk communication. As a result of poor communication to the public by the government the public lost trust in the government. This effect is inevitable in local government also, if the process of risk communication is not taken seriously.

The BSE crisis once again highlighted the differences between perceptions of those involved in managing the situation and the public. Although most of those concerned with handling BSE interpreted the available scientific evidence as indicating that the likelihood that BSE posed a risk was remote, they did not trust the public to adopt as sanguine an attitude. Ministers, officials and scientific advisory committees alike were all apprehensive that the public would react irrationally to BSE (Phillips Report 2000).

Finally, with regard to this issue, there is the role of the environmental health practitioner as an enforcer of food safety standards. Where government presented one view and the public an opposite view, environmental health practitioners were caught in the middle of the debate, as decisions concerning risk were being made at central government level. Eventually, the new government introduced legislation prohibiting the sale of beef on the bone and expected environmental health practitioners to enforce this law. Within a short period of time, it became apparent that this was an unpopular, unenforceable piece of legislation and it was eventually repealed.

It can be seen therefore that the BSE debate largely focussed around issues of scientific certainty. Whilst local authority environmental health practitioners were involved, to a large extent it was on the periphery of the debate. However, many communities and elected representatives were asking these somewhat marginalised professionals to comment on issues and provide some measure of reassurance to a constituency that was very much ill at ease.

Housing

This section provides a brief EHO perspective on aspects of housing that have been dealt with in the previous chapter (HMSO 1985). As well as dealing with complaints from residents of property about housing conditions, the key role of the environmental health service within the housing field is the determination of the suitability of property for occupation. The standard of fitness for human habitation (similar to the tolerable standard found in Scotland) is a set of basic requirements that dwelling houses should have in order to be considered as acceptable places to live. If a property fails one or more of the criteria listed within the standard, the local authority is under a duty to declare the dwelling house unfit for human habitation and take action with regard to the property. Such action usually involves requiring the owner to repair the property. In extreme circumstances the only options available may be to either prevent the house being used for occupation or to demolish the property.

During the late 1990s the government conducted research which utilised the growing body of knowledge on risk and risk assessment. The concern was to publish a new standard of fitness that reflects an understanding of the health and safety hazards and risks within dwellings. The Government consulted widely in 1998 via the Department of the Environment, Transport and the Regions (DETR 1998), and the initial findings of its research were published in July 2000 (DETR 2000a). They also published the first detailed guidance of the operation of the proposed Housing Health and Safety Rating System (HHSRS) (DETR 2000b).

The new system will allow local authority enforcement officers to measure the severity of the risks associated with any health and safety hazards in the dwelling, by referring to 24 broad categories of housing hazard. The condition of the property is first assessed visually, and a note is made, either electronically or on paper, of the actual faults found. There then follows a two-stage assessment of process. First, an assessment is made of which faults will contribute to hazards, and the severity of such a hazard. Second, the likelihood of an occurrence (such as an accident) is evaluated. An assessment is then made of the possible health outcomes of such an event. Combining these two factors gives a 'Hazard Profile Rating' for the premises, which can be directly related to an equivalent annual risk of death. In effect there is an attempt at a 'semi-quantitative' risk assessment of the premises.

The proposals are not without their critics. Parkinson and Fairman (2000) have extensively reviewed the proposed changes. They argue that whilst the intention is to provide an evidence-based methodology 'there is little sound evidence underlying it and it is a recipe for litigation' (Parkinson and Fairman 2000). They further argue that there is currently not enough data to allow an evidence-based quantitative risk assessment process to be realistically undertaken. Finally, they argue that the use of the Health and Safety Executive's (HSE) Tolerability of Risk Framework to produce benchmarks is misguided, pointing to the HSE's own decision to extensively promote gas safety in the home, even though the risks involved are far lower than calculated tolerability limits.

These criticisms elicited a speedy response from those involved in the development of the new system. In a follow-up article Ormandy *et al.* argue that there is a wealth of evidence to support the proposed changes (Ormandy *et al.* 2000). They point to Building Research Establishment Reports, DTI assessments of home accidents, and successive National House Condition Surveys. The new system, it is argued, therefore not only has a strong evidence base, but also allows for the development of further research on the relationship between housing conditions and health and safety risks.

Despite this ongoing debate, it would appear that the government is committed to change. Currently (2002) they are consulting on the range of enforcement options and enforcement mechanisms that should be available to local authorities after the introduction of the new Rating System (DETR 2001).

Air quality

The Environment Act 1995 required the government to develop a National Air Quality Strategy covering England, Wales, Scotland and Northern Ireland. The strategy was originally published in 1997 and revised in January 2000 (DETR 2000d).

Air pollution has been recognised as a serious public health problem which has been attributed to the premature death of over 20 000 people each year and the need for hospital treatment for many thousands of people each year, at a great cost to the National Health Service. A new type of invisible pollution has replaced the problems caused by the old urban smogs as a result of burning fossil fuels. This has been created to a large extent by the development of transport over the past three decades or so, as well as the significant contribution made by industrial processes and power generation. The National Air Quality Strategy sets targets for airborne levels of eight major air pollutants which are known to affect human health, including benzene, 1,3-butadiene, carbon monoxide, lead, nitrogen dioxide, ozone, PM10 particles and sulphur dioxide.

Local authorities are required to draw up their own strategies for achieving the air quality objectives in their own areas under the process known as Local Air Quality Management (LAQM). The monitoring, as well as general regulatory controls including the creation of smoke control areas, are undertaken by environmental health practitioners. Many local authorities display up-to-date air quality data from monitoring instruments in civic buildings and on internet sites, and there is an increasing application of modelling system in use, to predict air quality data over a wide geographical area.

Although the environmental health service is central to the gathering and analysis of data, certain activities such as those concerned with relieving traffic congestion are undertaken in conjunction with the planning authorities. Finally, education campaigns designed to get people to walk or use public transport are becoming an increasingly important aspect of the work of the environmental health department.

Water quality

The environmental health service is responsible for dealing with several different aspects of water quality, including drinking water from either mains supplies or private supplies and also recreational water supplies such as swimming pools and bathing water quality. These duties interlink with the responsibilities of other Central Government Agencies such as the Drinking Water Inspectorate and the Environment Agency.

Mains water is used by most dwellings in the United Kingdom as well as being used by a range of food manufacturers. Working in concert with the statutory water undertakers and the Drinking Water Inspectorate of the Department for Environment, Food and Rural Affairs (DEFRA) local authority environmental health practitioners undertake periodic sampling of mains supplies. Local authorities have a duty under the Water Industry Act 1991 (HMSO 1991) to ensure themselves that the water supplied to their area by statutory water undertakers is wholesome. They also monitor this by the regular examination of published monitoring data.

There is a variation between local authorities but in many, environmental health personnel will sample water from each water supply zone in their district. A sampling regime is developed to allow for samples to be taken on an annual basis. Samples are assessed independently against the key parameters laid down in the Water Supply (Water Quality) Regulations 1989 (HMSO 1989). It is perhaps interesting to note that some local authorities even sample the water quality from drinking water fountains, to ensure that consumers are protected.

With regard to private water supplies from wells, springs and boreholes, serving either domestic or commercial premises, the local authority are the responsible authority for ensuring that the supplies are satisfactory from both a microbiological and a chemical (e.g. pesticides) point of view. Testing frequencies are laid down in regulations.

The 11th Annual Report of the Drinking Water Inspectorate (DEFRA 2000) shows that the results obtained are the best so far, as almost 100 per cent of the 2.7 million water samples taken met the appropriate quality standards.

Recreational water supplies such as private swimming pools in hotels and fitness clubs are regularly monitored by environmental health practitioners as part of their public health regime. Such pools can be the source of infection which can give rise to a range of eye, ear and skin complaints. Testing is carried out on a regular basis to ensure that such pools comply with the guidelines set down by DEFRA and the Public Health Laboratory Service (PHLS).

One additional potential public health problem which is associated with both drinking water and recreational waters is the appearance of a protozoan parasite known as Cryptosporidium. Ingesting the oocysts of this organism results in a set of symptoms commonly associated with food-borne disease, which can last for 30 days or more in healthy adults. Annual notifications of cases of

Cryptosporidium continue to increase from year to year, and in 2000, the figure reached 7000 (PHLS 2001). Environmental health practitioners are frequently involved in the sampling of water supplies as part of an outbreak control team, as in the case of food-borne disease (CIEH 1997).

With regard to bathing waters, coastal local authorities tend to take regular samples of seawater which are analysed by the PHLS during the bathing season between May and September each year to supplement samples taken by the Environment Agency. Samples are tested for compliance with the standards prescribed in the European Community Directive on Bathing Water Quality (Directive 76/106/EEC). Results are often published on beaches and also on local authority websites for the information of prospective bathers.

It must be recognised that compliance with the Directive is often of economic importance as the results will influence tourism levels via the award of a range of bathing beach award schemes.

In summary therefore, the range of water quality issues illustrated above, demonstrate that environmental health practitioners have a key role in undertaking monitoring and analysis of samples, and communicating the results, along with appropriate explanations, to the local community. Whilst the risks involved may appear to be minor, the influence on the public health status of the local population is significant. Local environmental health services have often been instrumental in calling for improvements in the standards of either drinking water or bathing water in an area.

Best Value and target setting

The role of any local government agency cannot be discussed without at least a brief reference to the topic of Best Value. The Local Government Act 1999 (HMSO 1999c) requires local authorities to consult with the community as part of their Best Value regime, this aims to help show the authority if the services which they provide are effective and are what the public actually wants. Also the Local Government Act 2000 (HMSO 2000b) requires the local authority to consult with the local community in relation to implementing a community action plan.

One of the problems associated with traditional models of service delivery is that they can be driven purely or mainly by performance targets. There is an assumption that, for example, achieving minimum numbers of traditional inspections of premises will have an effective impact upon environmental factors and thereby have a positive impact upon public health.

It is interesting to reflect on the findings of recent research undertaken on behalf of the HSE (HSE 2000). Here a number of qualified and experienced environmental health practitioners were asked to attribute inspection rating scores for a series of premises, as a desktop exercise. The resulting scores, by which inspection frequency can be prioritised, demonstrated a very wide range, for every type of premises examined. This type of research raises questions concerning the objectivity of the process in question. Furthermore, the validity of routine inspections of individual premises as a tool for protecting the public might then be questioned. This is particularly of concern, for example, when numbers of inspections are set as performance criteria by organisations such as the FSA acting under the influence of the European Commission.

What this type of evidence implies is that inspection by environmental health practitioners is merely one of the instruments that can be used. It seems clear that, in order to create and establish a sustainable model for the creation and enhancement of a new public health model, that consideration needs to be given to the adoption of a wide range of methodologies and involvement of a variety of partners.

The environmental health practitioner in the community

When considering the input of the environmental health practitioner into the various processes designed to protect public health, the question of trust between stakeholders is an important consideration. Frewer (1999) argues that 'Who trusts whom and why' is potentially one of the most important issues in risk communication. If central or local government is to effectively communicate the risks associated with different hazards, it is essential that the importance of source characteristics as potential influences on risk communication effectiveness be understood.

The Department of Health (1997) states that in most circumstances, messages are judged first and foremost not by content but by source: Members of the public will often ask themselves, 'who is telling me this, and can I trust them?' If the answer to the second question is no, then any message is liable to be disregarded, no matter how well intentioned and well delivered. Perhaps the most important constituent of trust is therefore not content but source. The simple message is that if we do not trust the source then we will not trust the message (Pidgeon *et al.* 1992). Indeed, there is even some evidence that well-presented arguments from distrusted sources actually have a negative effect (DoH 1997). The Department of Health goes on to say that there is a general decline in trust in scientific expertise and argue that reliance on scientific credentials alone is therefore unlikely to work.

Environmental health practitioners must therefore communicate to both the public and elected representatives in a way they can relate to. Technical language and jargon, whilst useful within a professional context, prevent effective communication with the community. Risk comparisons may well be used by some professionals to put risks into perspective (DoH 1997), but these same professionals must acknowledge people's perceptions and note the differences between those and those of the experts.

In many cases the environmental health practitioner is closely involved in mediating between the various stakeholders associated with issues affecting the public's health. For example, when plans are put forward for the development of land for commercial or industrial use it is often the environmental health practitioner who is seen as being able to present an impartial opinion. It is they who should be able to interpret technical information and communicate its contents to the wider public. In order to do this they must obtain the trust, not only of the public, but also of the developers. Herein lies the dilemma for the environmental health practitioner. How can they be seen as the honest broker by all parties?

The Local Government Management Board in its paper *Involving the Public* (1998) recommends approaches that local authorities can use to involve the public such as user panels, focus groups, citizens' groups, referenda, open evenings, surveys and area meetings. Similar approaches can, and in some cases are, adapted to forge links with commercial and industrial interests. For example, some local authorities have established industry liaison groups to discuss approaches to compliance with air quality guidelines. Similar groups have been established to involve landlords of residential property in discussing approaches for the improvement of housing standards. In this way, it is considered that practitioners can win the trust of all parties, and seek to ensure that messages are clearly understood. Such an approach to the involvement of all stakeholders is embodied within the Local Government Act 2000. Here there is a requirement for local authorities to develop Community Strategies that include consultation and involvement of not only the local community, but also the business community.

In seeking to attain this role of honest broker, the involvement of other agencies by environmental health practitioners can be effective, particularly when it comes to communicating risk information. Public conflict with other credible sources may prove destructive (Covello 1998). If the public does not trust the local authority then the authority may be able to form alliances with more credible sources such as the local health authority (ILGRA 1998). In addition, local authorities can form alliances with other agencies or groups not just to gain credibility but also to gain valuable experience and expertise. For example, environmental groups may have more experience in communicating about environmental risks than the local authority. Local authorities can also consult with councillors or other elected representatives to help gain public trust, or even use the trustworthy source as a spokesperson (Covello 1998).

Skills for the future

This process of the communication of risks in order to secure improvements in public health, may question the skills of environmental health practitioners. Even if they have those skills there is an assumption that the local government environment will allow them to flourish.

The above text demonstrates the wide range of abilities required to undertake the functions of an environmental health department. The question must be put as to whether the profession is properly equipped for the future. To answer this point, recent survey was undertaken by the Local Government National Training Organisation (LGNTO) between November 2000 and March 2001 (LGNTO 2001). In their research, LGNTO carried out in-depth interviews with environmental health practitioners working in ten local authorities.

The research recognised that such personnel undertake a wide range of functions in a set of diverse fields of work. In summary, the study determined that environmental health practitioners have coped and adapted to the changes in local authorities and in general terms there are few problems associated with a skills gap. It is worthy of note that the view obtained from the officers surveyed was one of uncertainty regarding the lack of control which such officers have over the future. The Best Value regime is perceived to have created a system where multiple-function inspections are combined in the interests of cost-saving and efficiency. Whilst the skills gaps identified were few, the area of specific personnel and project management training were identified.

Conclusions

The above discussion has served to highlight that the modern day environmental health practitioner is a well-trained, professional officer with a range of scientific, technical, social and legal skills, which can be brought together, to secure significant improvements in public health via the process of assessing and managing risks. These skills are particularly effective when combined with other stakeholders at community level.

Overall, the profession has developed its longstanding role and acquired new skills as necessary, to address new public health issues. However, to conclude on a warning note, Agendas for Change reminds us that 'We are, in effect, driving an old vehicle into a new era. Do we leave it to creak along, attempting the odd roadside repair, or send it back to the design shop for a complete overhaul?' (CIEH 1997).

References

Burningham K and Thrush D (2001) *Rainforests are a Long Way from Here, the Environmental Concerns of Disadvantaged Groups.* Joseph Rowntree Foundation.

Centre for Environmental Sciences (1999) *Going for Green Sustainable Communities Project,* Volumes 1–5. University of Wales Institute, Cardiff.

Chartered Institute of Environmental Health (CIEH) (1997) *Commission for Environmental Health*. Agendas for Change, Chadwick House Group Ltd.

Covello V, Sandman P and Slovic P (1988) *Risk Communication, Risk Statistics and Risk Comparisons: A Manual for Plant Managers*. Chemical Manufacturers Association, Washington, DC.

Covello VT (1998) 'Risk communication' in Calow (ed.) *Handbook of Environmental Risk Assessment and Management*. Blackwell Science, London.

Department of Health (1997) Communicating about risks to public health – pointers to good practice. HMSO, London.

Department of Environment (1994) *Planning Policy Guidance: Planning and Pollution Control*. PPG23.

Department of the Environment, Transport and the Regions (1998) *Housing Fitness Standard*. Consultation Paper.

Department of the Environment, Transport and the Regions (2000a) *Housing Health and Safety Rating System*. Report and Development.

Department of the Environment, Transport and the Regions (2000b) *Housing Health and Safety Rating System*. The Guidance (Version 1).

Department of the Environment, Transport and the Regions (2000c) *Guidelines for Environmental Risk Assessment and Management*. Revised Departmental Guidance.

Department of the Environment, Transport and the Regions (2000d) *The Air Quality Strategy for England, Scotland, Wales and Northern Ireland: Working Together for Clean Air*.

Department of the Environment, Transport and the Regions (2001) *Health and Safety in Housing*. A Consultation Paper.

Department for the Environment, Food and Rural Affairs (2000) *Drinking Water 2000 – A Report by the Chief Inspector*. 11th Annual Report of the Drinking Water Inspectorate.

Food Standards Agency (2001) *Strategy for Wider Implementation of HACCP*. Paper FSA 01/07/02, 14 November.

Frewer LJ (1999) 'Public risk perceptions and risk communication' in Bennett P and Calman K (eds) *1999 Risk Communication and Public Health*. Oxford University Press, Oxford.

Groth E (1991) Communicating with consumers about food safety and risk issues. *Food Tech* **45**(5): 248–53.

Gowman N and Coote A (2000) *Evidence and Public Health – Towards a Common Framework*. Kings Fund.

HMSO (1985) *Housing Act 1985*.

HMSO (1989) *The Water Supply (Water Quality) Regulations 1989*.

HMSO (1991) *The Water Industry Act 1991*.

HMSO (1999a) *Saving Lives – Our Healthier Nation*. Government White Paper.

HMSO (1999b) *The Control of Major Accident Hazard Regulations 1999*.

HMSO (1999c) *Local Government Act 1999.*

HMSO (2000a) *The National Health Service Plan – A Plan for Investment – A Plan for Reform.*

HMSO (2000b) *The Local Government Act 2000.*

Health and Safety Executive (HSE) (2000) *An Analysis of the Application of HELA Circular 67/1 (revised) by Local Authorities and the Development of Indicative Hazard/Risk Scores for Generic Premises Types.* Contract Research Report 297/2000.

Inter-departmental Liaison Group on Risk Assessment (ILGRA) (1998) *Risk Communication – A Guide to Regulatory Practice.* HSE.

Kasperson RE, Renn O, Slovic P *et al.* (1988) The social amplification of risk: a conceptual framework. *Risk Analysis* **6**: 177.

Local Government Management Board (LGMB) (1998) *Involving the public.* LGMB.

Local Government National Training Organisation (LGNTO) (2001) *Skills for the Future – Environmental Health Officers.* LGNTO.

McArthur I (2001) The Agenda has changed. *Environ Health J.* October.

Ormandy D, Moore R and Battersby S (2000) If it's broke, fix it fully. *Environ Health J,* December.

Parkinson N and Fairman R (2000) If it ain't broke, don't fix it. *Environ Health J,* October.

Phillips Report (2000) *BSE Enquiry Report.* HMSO.

Public Health Laboratory Service (PHLS) (2001) www.phls.co.uk

Pidgeon N, Hood C, Jones D, Turner B and Gibson R (1992) 'Risk perception' in The Royal Society (1992 publication) *Risk: Analysis, Perception and Management.* The Royal Society Group, London.

Renn O and Levine D (1991) 'Credibility and trust in risk communication' in Kasperson RE and Stallen PJM (eds) *Communicating Risks to the Public.* Kluwer, Dordrecht, pp 175–210.

Slovic P (1987) Perception of risk. *Science* **236**: 280–5.

Smith D and McCloskey J (1998) Risk communication and the social amplification of public sector risk. *Public Money and Management* **18**(4): 41–50.

The Royal Society (1992) *Risk: Analysis, Perception and Management.* The Royal Society, London.

Welsh Office (1998) *Better Health Better Wales.* A Consultation Paper.

9

Occupational Health

Andrew Watterson

Introduction

Work should ideally contribute to good health and wellbeing as well as to individual and national economic prosperity. All too often and for all too many people especially in developing countries it does not. Employees are threatened by a wide range of physical, biological, chemical, work organisation and psychosocial hazards in their work that lead to a heavy toll of occupationally caused and occupationally related ill-health. That is why commentators have described the modern workplace as a battlefield with casualties that have often exceeded those in major wars. The public health consequences of such large-scale mortality and morbidity are considerable.

This chapter will briefly look at the scale of the problem and how occupationally caused and occupationally related diseases and accidents form part of the public health challenge (Box 9.1). It will then focus on how occupational health and safety practitioners may and do intervene to prevent such diseases and accidents. The barriers that prevent good practice will be analysed. Finally, the best solutions available to promote good occupational health and safety standards in the workplace will be examined.

Box 9.1   Problems with UK occupational health and safety

Large-scale toll of UK workforce in disease and accidents.

Lack of enforcement, linked to deregulation, to raise occupational health and safety standards.

Overemphasis on cultural and behavioural factors in workplace health and safety.

Lack of focus in the past on labour trend changes and workplace organisations that impact upon occupational health and safety, neglect or ignorance of problems created by psychosocial and physical stresses, aggressive and poor management.

Resources lacking for work health and safety in government and business services.

Lack of adequate data about size, distribution and causation of diseases and accidents.

Lack of detailed sectoral, gender and ethnicity analyses of workplace health and safety.

Lack of full disclosure of information on hazards and risks relating to workplaces.

Lack of commitment to ensuring corporate accountability in this field.

Unbalanced approach to risk management that has led to a neglect of hazard identification and removal as the first step in successful health and safety strategies.

Inability now or in the past to action effective precautionary principle strategies to control such problems as chemicals including endocrine disrupters, asbestos and other carcinogens and reproductive health hazards.

Failure to link effectively workplace and wider environmental hazard actions.

Failure to use resources of trade unions and communities to act against known and potential hazards.

Table 9.1 documents the toll taken in UK workplaces by occupational and occupationally related ill-health (Box 9.2). It also indicates major gaps in our knowledge or areas of uncertainty about the effects of some exposures.

The public health challenge

This is an enormous public health challenge although it is not always recognised as such and may be marginalised by politicians and policy makers who often reflect employer rather than

Table 9.1   Estimates of occupational ill-health in UK in 1990s

1. 2 million adults with illnesses believe those illnesses are caused or made worse by work causing 18 million lost working days (HSE 2001a).
2. 10% of General Practitioner consultations are work-related (Sheffield Occupational Health Project figure).
3. Conservative estimates indicate up to 6% of cancers are caused each year by workplace exposures and 6% of cancers may have workplace exposures as contributory factors. Others estimate at least 12% or more of cancer deaths could be occupationally related. 12 000 occupational cancer deaths per year with at least 5000 coming from asbestos is quite possible. 5 million GB workers or 22% of the workforce are estimated to be exposed to carcinogens excluding asbestos and agro-chemicals (Hazards 2000: 13).
4. HSC estimated that there were at least 2000 premature deaths each year from occupational disease, 8000 deaths each year where work contributed to the mortality at least 80 000 new cases of work-related disease each year with more than 500 000 people suffering continuing damage to health from work.
5. Asbestos-related deaths estimated in the 1980s by HSE and epidemiologists is likely to be at least 2000 a year with up to 50 000 deaths occurring between 1982 and 2012 at TLVs set for asbestos in the early 1980s. These figures are recognised as significant underestimates. Deaths among workers from exposure to asbestos will treble over the next 20 years and deaths per year may total up to 9000 a year by 2020.
6. UK SWORD (Surveillance of work-related occupational respiratory diseases) – which is investigating occupationally related respiratory diseases suggests that there may be three times the number of such diseases occurring as is reported. These are probably gross underestimates of the true damage done to workers by occupationally related respiratory diseases. Up to a third of all US adult asthma cases may be caused or exacerbated by exposure to chemicals, dust or fumes in the work environment. At least 20% of all UK asthma cases are estimated to be work-related. 68 000 workers in the United Kingdom are estimated to be affected by workplace asthma.
7. 426 000 workers in the United Kingdom use tools which expose them to hand/arm vibration and 152 000 use such equipment for relatively long periods. In 1988–89 1056 vibration-induced whitefinger cases received benefit in Britain. It is estimated that some 30 000 are suffering now from vibration-induced whitefinger (VWF).
8. HSE estimate 50 000 cases of self-reported Repetitive Strain Injury (RSI) in the country. Finland estimated that 53% of butchers had carpal tunnel syndrome. 18% of Swedish scissors makers and 56% of Swedish packers had tendon lesions. 1996 New Labour Force Survey estimates

1.5 million cases of musculo-skeletal injuries each year in the United Kingdom: with backs the major cause of injury and RSIs next in importance.

9. No accurate data or even guesstimates exist for occupationally caused and related neurological diseases in the United Kingdom. Current OP and painters solvent poisoning cases indicate that we are seeing just the tip of a national iceberg. 2.5 million workers estimated to be exposed to solvents in the United Kingdom. 10 000 cases of solvent dementia per year are estimated in the United Kingdom.

10. No data exist for cardio-vascular illnesses caused by work. HSE estimated 45 100 work related cases of heart diseases, hypertension and stroke. Chemicals, physical hazards, biological hazards, dust, metals and occupational stress may all be factors here. In the United States 26% of cardio-vascular diseases may be occupationally linked.

11. Immune system damage – no data/no estimates are available. Links between occupational exposures and diseases do exist with regard to vinyl chloride monomer (VCM) and various solvents as well as specific health service hazards.

12. HSE 1993 study 104 900 occupational stress cases estimated in England and Wales alone. In 1996, the new Labour Force survey estimates 300 000 cases of workers psychologically affected by work with 160 000 cases of health-related stress symptoms – including heart disease – reported.

employee interests (Watterson, 2001). Public health debates about social exclusion and health inequalities have rarely focused on occupational health and safety. Most cancer policies focus on screening and treatment and neglect prevention policies that must involve occupational health even when mesotheliomas and lung cancers due to asbestos exposure provide a significant fraction of cancer mortality figures. In the United Kingdom and Northern Ireland for instance between 1997 and 2001, 18 000 people have died from all asbestos diseases (Tudor 2001: 4).

Additionally, in recent years, numerous reports in the United Kingdom, Australia and the United States produced by government economists and academics have shown that poor health and safety is a major financial burden for any society. In the United Kingdom as much as one full year of increased economic growth may be lost – up to £7 billion – due to occupational accidents and ill-health. Individual workers so injured in 1995/96 were estimated

Box 9.2   The Global and European scale of the problem

Late 1990s – Around 2600 million people in the global workforce
Three quarters of this number in developing countries
Each year around 40 million people join that labour force.
ILO and WHO estimate – 250 million occupational injuries each year
– 160 million cases of occupational disease globally each year
– 10 million workplace accidents occur in Europe each year
Well known, well established, well tried and tested and often simple preventive measures exist to reduce these figures significantly.
30% of the workforce in developed countries and 70% of the workforce in developed countries face major ergonomic hazards.

In industrialised countries, ergonomic problems are the major cause of short-term disability and job loss and can account for up to 5% of a nation's GNP. Solutions to such problems may exist: they do not require 'rocket science'.

200 world-wide biological hazards including asthmagens and viruses.

3000 allergenic substances in use in workplaces.

350 chemicals have been identified already as occupational carcinogens.

16 million workers are exposed to carcinogenic substances (WHO 1996).

100 000 different chemicals used in the twenty-first century workplace.

Asbestos in Europe between 1999 and 2034 will cause an estimated 250 000 deaths from the asbestos-caused mesothelioma (Peto *et al.* 1999). Others estimate two asbestos-related lung cancer deaths for every one mesothelioma death producing a million deaths in the same period in Europe from just two types of cancer caused by asbestos (Hazards 1999: 1–2).

Scientific/medical/engineering knowledge has existed for well over a 100 years to tackle the asbestos problem but has often not been used (Castleman 1996).

to have lost £558 million in reduced income and additional expenditure at 1995/96 prices (HSE 2001a). The burden also includes physical and emotional costs not just to individuals but to families and communities. These are public health concerns too but the support given to individuals by medical, nursing, social services may be relatively small and is sometimes non-existent in the fields of welfare benefits, rehabilitation and employment opportunities. These fields are a critical part of occupational health and safety yet they are rarely addressed by occupational health and safety practitioners. Workplace health and safety has been effectively marginalised for many decades in the United Kingdom although the recent Revitalising Health and Safety programme of Health and Safety Executive (HSE) and the report of the Health and Safety Commission's (HSC) Occupational Health Advisory Committee have proposed a more integrated and holistic approach to the whole subject (DETR 2001; OHAC 2002). NHS Plus, floated in 2000, now has a network of 100 NHS occupational health departments that sell their services to private companies. They also provide information for employers about occupational health management and legal standards. HSE too are now looking at how changes in work patterns and employment in the United Kingdom may affect health and safety and such policy and research developments will help to inform occupational health and safety practitioners better.

Cutting ill-health at work is a financially cost-effective measure if total costs to individuals, communities and society are considered although those creating hazards may offload or lose the costs on society as a whole. This is because the principle of 'the employer pays full legal, economic, medical and social costs for damaging the health and safety of employees' does not yet operate. Estimates exist of as many as 25 000 UK workers each year losing jobs due to work-related disability (Hazards 2000: 18–19).

Effective occupational health policies and practices appear to be absent in many Health Action Zones (HAZ) and health improvement plans in the United Kingdom. It is likely to be marginalised even further in English primary care group and trust priorities although perhaps less so in Scotland. HAZ in some places such as Sandwell described in Chapter 4 are trying to address these issues but their effectiveness has yet to be demonstrated. The impacts of poor health and safety on primary and acute health services are substantial in terms of bed occupancy, the problems of treating acute and chronic workplace illnesses and accidents, the time spent by nurses, GPs, physiotherapists, surgeons and physicians. These are again public health issues. To save money, make industry more efficient, productive and environmentally safe and improve public health, we need better occupational health standards, practices and services in the United Kingdom. Ensuring good health and safety standards may also prevent catastrophic financial failures of some companies because of occupational disease or accident compensation costs.

The figures reveal that in some workplace settings, we know about certain hazards, we understand the risks and can take effective action to remove those risks. Interventions have occurred but the statistics demonstrate that much work is still required to reduce the avoidable toll of disease and injury. In other areas, our knowledge of disease mechanisms, multiple exposures, low level exposures and so on is incomplete. This is why some occupational health and safety practitioners argue that it is essential we should learn from our past mistakes and build in a precautionary approach to dealing with uncertain hazards and unknown risks (EEA 2001).

How occupational health and safety practitioners may and do intervene

Effective occupational health and safety practice requires technical skills, power to influence workplace organisation and production and financial decisions and an ability to liaise with a wide variety of agencies. Occupational health and safety practitioners may include occupational health and safety advisors, occupational health and safety managers, risk managers, occupational or industrial hygienists, occupational health nurses, occupational physicians, safety engineers and other engineers, occupational psychologists and ergonomists (Ladou 1997). They may also include trade union safety representatives and safety engineers found active unions to be the single most important factor in delivering safety improvements (Abrams 2001). As there are 200 000 safety reps in the United Kingdom and some 25 000 IOSH members, the former offer an enormous health and safety resource that should be used far better by government and in workplaces.

All the above groups have an important part to play in the contribution of occupational health and safety to better public health and they demonstrate the truly multi-disciplinary and sometimes inter-disciplinary nature of the subject. The chapter focuses on what might be termed the occupational health and safety advisor or practitioner – sometimes called the safety engineer in North America – who would bring together knowledge of or expertise in occupational health, occupational hygiene, toxicology and epidemiology, safety engineering, law and risk management. They are the largest professional occupational health and safety group in the United Kingdom with some 25 000 members. Effective action in this field requires technical knowledge and skills and negotiating and communication skills and all are mediated by legal, economic and political factors.

Central to their practice is the development, implementation and audit of health and safety policies within their organisations. This is illustrated below by the HSE's classic feedback loop of the early 1990s.

The occupational health and safety professional to be fully effective therefore needs to bring managerial, technical, process, political and economic bargaining skills to bear within and outside workplaces. This creates real tensions between such professionals, employers, employees and sometimes communities: they may be advocates of good practice, overseers of minimum standards or instruments for the organisations within which they work. Sometimes and on some issues they may wear different hats and take different positions. Typically they develop and update health and safety systems and audit and review 'safety' policies with the aim of getting such policies recognised and supported throughout the organisation. They may also contribute to or lead the development of appropriate health and safety management structures, unambiguous means of health and safety control, adequate resourcing and effective communication and coordination between all relevant sections of the organisation.

Planning through setting and progressing of health and safety objectives listed above is the critical issue. Hazard removal rather than risk management should be the first step. When faced with a number of hazards which require simultaneous assessment and control, items to be tackled immediately should be identified and decisions regarding priorities should be addressed in a plan. Again this may be a source of tension and conflict or require skilful advocacy as may the implementation and monitoring of plans and measurement of performance. Active systems are needed to confirm the compliance with specific good or best practice

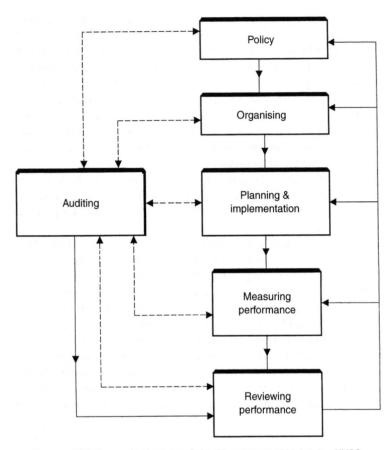

Source: HSE, Successful Health and Safety Management, 1991. London: HMSO.

requirements established in the plan, and reactive systems which seek to analyse the impact of unplanned events such as accidents and ill-health (Watterson and Wright 1998). Health and safety professionals may frequently lack access to disease data or be unable to produce a complete and coherent 'public health' response to threats to health and safety in their workplaces.

The HSE identified long ago a range of key activities for health and safety managers (HSE Successful Health and Safety Management 1991 and amended) which in practice can relate to a minimalist rather than a good practice role for such practitioners. Activities included strategic and tactical, organisational as well as technical roles. For instance in helping formulate and develop policies; to help structure and operate the health and safety organisation and systems; to plan short-term, middle-term and long-term health and safety objectives and to prioritise those objectives; to develop performance standards for the objectives set; to implement the systems established on a day-to-day basis and to monitor and analyse policy and plans and performance. Other tasks would entail maintaining adequate information systems both legal and technical; interpreting and applying the relevant health and safety laws in the workplace setting; investigating accidents, occupational diseases, near misses and important health and safety problems; and liaising with employees about health and safety.

The barriers to good practice and effective action in occupational health and safety – an asbestos case study

This small case study explores how occupational health and safety practitioners may address a problem at different levels and in different ways. Asbestos has been widely used across the globe for many centuries. Its properties made it a valuable industrial and commercial commodity and little was known about its toxicity until the end of the nineteenth century and the beginning of twentieth century. The United Kingdom played a major role in the early twentieth century through toxicologists, chest physicians, hygienists and trade unions in exposing the health effects of the 'magic mineral'. Yet, asbestos in all its forms causes serious lung diseases such as asbestosis and several types of cancer including lung cancer and mesothelioma.

In 1897, the Austrian physician Netoliszky described the respiratory illnesses of asbestos weavers, recognised that asbestos dust was the cause and called for wet processing methods and ventilation. In 1906 Auribault in France reported 16 deaths from pulmonary fibrosis in a French asbestos textile factory and this was also followed by calls for better ventilation controls and respirators (Castleman 1996). These solutions were ones that occupational health and safety practitioners could implement. Such action would, however, be conditional on having sufficient information, having the support of the company or organisation to take action against asbestos and this would be partly determined by regulations and laws in effect to control, remove or cease to purchase asbestos.

At an international level asbestos bans have now been introduced with regard to the purchase, manufacture and use of new asbestos products and materials. Hence, a key activity of the health and safety practitioners would be to keep abreast of these developments and ensure that employers and employees were informed. Second, such professionals would need to be aware of the purchasing policy of their organisation and know which new products contained asbestos and which did not. Third, where asbestos exposure could still occur in the workplace through existing asbestos materials, arrangements would need to be in place with a strategy if possible to prevent exposure and remove the asbestos including safe disposal as well as to ensure where necessary employee health was monitored if exposures had occurred. Fourth, policies on asbestos removal and control standards would be needed. There might be minimum legal standards and the issue for the health and safety professional would be – what is best health and safety practice; what is acceptable professional practice; what is minimum legally acceptable practice? Pressures from employers on the professional as an employee would then come to bear and influence the outcome. Health and safety professionals may find conflicting tensions described earlier operating – duties to the organisation, duties to the workforce, duties to line managers, legal accountability, ethical accountability and moral concerns may impinge on the judgement. The time, resources, cost, technical difficulty, process or activity disruption pressures may all come into play.

The risks to contractors and sub-contractors as well as employees and potential risks to communities where asbestos may exist in public buildings, housing, facilities open to the public all require addressing. The debate between sealing in asbestos products or removing them presents the health and safety practitioner with perhaps the most demanding challenge especially when the material may be present in large quantities in hospitals, theatres, cinemas, swimming baths, schools, colleges and houses and may be damaged in situ. The hazard removal, risk assessment and management, risk communication, cost–benefit analyses required of the occupational health and safety practitioner in these settings are considerable, complex and problematic. The line between occupational health, environmental health and public health is also very blurred when dealing with asbestos because it presents threats to all three.

The professional barriers – roles and challenges

There may be a strategic and policy bias to the work of an occupational health and safety professional working at board level or in a non-governmental organisation (NGO) or at a national level in a trade union; a tactical approach for a company or workplace health and safety advisor or regional trade union health advisor; a technical role for an industrial hygienist, engineer or trade union safety representative monitoring dust, fumes, noise, lighting and other shopfloor problems. Labour or government health and safety inspectors tend to concentrate on information, advice and enforcement work within the constraints of legislation and governmental policy on occupational hazards and risks.

In many parts of Western Europe, there are Labour inspectors who have a role on welfare and working conditions as well as workplace hazards: this is not the case in the United Kingdom with the HSE. In small- and medium-sized enterprises where there may be a very small number of staff, busy managers will find that they need to add occupational health and safety roles to their other activities. Globally it is estimated that there are about 10 000 million people working in small-scale industries. In the United Kingdom sometimes such groups and larger organisations too will use part-time health and safety advisors, occupational health services or consultants (WHO 1997).

With a range of different professional practitioner groups, not often found to the same extent within other areas of public health, there is potential for conflict, overlap or inactivity. Some of these matters have been addressed by the professional body for occupational health and safety practitioners – Institution of Occupational Safety and Health (IOSH: Professionals in Partnership 2001). This approach is supported by occupational health nurses, occupational hygienists, ergonomists, occupational physicians and HSE. There are also concerns for all health professional groups that practitioners function within their areas of competence and critically know their limits. This may be very difficult for those individuals and small teams where effective governance has not been properly developed or possibly may be absent and, if one does not know one's limits, one will not be able to recognise them. It may be a particular problem for consultants. Education, mentoring continuing professional development may all help address the problem.

There may also be real tensions within a particular occupational health and safety post. What happens when the interests of one group come into conflict with another? What happens when there are insufficient funds to address occupational health and safety deficiencies? What happens when budgets are set and managers are penalised for spending on occupational health and safety improvements as this may come out of a section budget but not penalised for accidents and diseases which come out of a central budget? What happens when a health and safety practitioner working for a multi-national company or organisations has to confront the operation of different standards on occupational health in different countries? These are major challenges especially in some regions, for instance Asia, Africa and Central and Eastern Europe where inward investment in plant may occur precisely because such things as occupational health and safety will be neglected or ignored (ECOHSE 2002).

What happens when profits or processes are put before the health and safety of the workforce? These issues have been explored at a macro and micro level and can be both simple and complex. For instance, the explosion on the Piper Alpha oil rig in the North Sea which killed 167 oil workers revealed that management at that time had 'maintained an exclusive prerogative over issues of safety, which was matched only by their determination to retain exclusive control over the work process....' (Woolfson *et al.* 1996: xix). The position of safety managers and worker representatives, if they exist, in such settings is difficult if not impossible as production demands and other pressures may override safety considerations. Similar problems emerged with Union Carbide Bhopal in India and with Thor in South Africa and Exxon in Australia (O'Neill 2002).

Dealing with such conflicts is helped by the provision of professional codes of conduct or ethics for most occupational health and safety professionals but this does not remove the problem. For instance, recent investigations have revealed fragmentation and poor management of the UK railway system. Track maintenance was neglected and the industry was chronically under-funded for many years. This benefited the shareholders but not the commuters or rail staff themselves and presented enormous difficulties for health and professionals working within the industry or responsible for its inspection and enforcement of the health and safety laws. How could health and safety professionals ensure adequate investment and rapid action to maintain basic health and safety standards? Who determines what is 'adequate investment', 'rapid action' and 'basic health and safety standards'? These matters will be the subject for negotiation within a legal, ethical and technical framework. The HSE's railway inspectorate has been found to be overloaded in the recent past, to lack rigour and to be somewhat gullible in accepting railway industry assurances about health and safety standards. The problems of being a health and safety practitioner in an under-funded industry which was fragmented and where shareholders and not employees and customers were regarded as the most important stakeholders would be exceptionally difficult.

Some have suggested that the whistleblowers charter will be the answer in the United Kingdom. Protection from victimisation for raising health at work concerns is important and many whistleblowers could come from the ranks of workplace health and safety. However, the effectiveness of such measures is still very unclear and other measures may be of far greater assistance in addressing major health and safety problems. A better approach would be to adopt codes of conduct that safeguarded practitioner, employees and in the process employers (LaDou *et al.* 2001). Recent international cases have demonstrated the need for such codes with the ending of the contract of an academic occupational physician in the United States who reported on new lung diseases in a research project on synthetic textile workers, and pressure put on a labour inspector in Brazil who pressed for asbestos bans as the most appropriate way of dealing with asbestos hazards.

Systems of work, compensation and insurance schemes and ethics play as much a part in occupational health and safer as toxicology and occupational medicine. What is viewed as inevitable, even timeless, for one occupational group in terms of accidents and ill-health would be totally unacceptable in another setting.

Problem solving and rule following

There is a tension between having a problem solving and rule following approach in occupational health and safety and how the two approaches can be brought together to produce effective and where necessary quick solutions. There are also tensions between wishing to integrate good health and safety practice into management practice and diluting health and safety because the professionals advise the managers and their advice may or may not be accepted and then implemented depending upon large and small economic, political, legal, cultural, organisational matters. This reflects the power and influence of the different parties.

One's employer may also determine the health and safety professional's response. For instance an HSE Inspector will work within a framework of rules, laws and guidance determined by the organisation: a senior health and safety advisor in a large multi-national where there are major health and safety hazards and risks may have more power and autonomy to effect change. A heavily regulated and frequently inspected large industry in the public eye will respond to health and safety pressures more quickly and have far more resources and staff at hand than an SME which may never be inspected and where staff would lack knowledge, time, resources, skills and systems to deal with many health and safety problems.

The old and limited model of health and safety practice was to ensure that laws such as the Factories Act 1961, the Mines and Quarries Act 1954, the Offices, Shops and Railway premises Act 1963 were enforced. These were rule followers who often simply saw occupational health and safety as safety and the major source of data and activity was a monthly lost-time accident report. There was little or no risk assessment and risk management and systems set up were rigid and inflexible. However, minimum legal standards were clear and easily enforced.

Now there is a greater emphasis on thinking critically within the health and safety profession and looking at responsive and flexible health and safety management approaches to solve problems. For some this has even gone so far as to advocate minimum standards, restricted enforcement and primarily voluntary approaches if not deregulation for health, safety and environmental matters. Unfortunately such models as the UK Robens system of self-regulation and joint regulation of health and safety have not necessarily proved successful. Recent UK enquiries have found, for example, that even where inspectorates existed they may have lacked rigour and proved gullible when told by management that health and safety standards and practices were good. There is a need to move from simple rule following to problem solving in occupational health and safety as well as environmental fields but such developments need to be underpinned by strong laws, good standards and effective enforcement. Research on these matters is lacking globally.

The work of the occupational health and safety practitioner in the twenty-first century now includes far greater emphasis on occupational health and, for many, a significant amount of work on environmental risk management, environmental monitoring systems and environmental pollution control issues. The need to bring together work environment issues with wider environmental issues and to control their interaction is now widely recognised. At a community, regional or national level, failures to address one often leads to failures to address the other. Planning to deal with environmental transitions is critical for health and safety practitioners in the context of the sunsetting of hazardous chemicals or the use of toxic-use reduction strategies to deal with high-risk substances or processes and replace them with lower risk materials. Ensuring sustainable jobs is also a key way of ensuring best health and safety practice.

Best practice solutions – using research and information

The science/professional interface

There may be a gulf between researchers and practitioners in terms of disseminating information and looking at how research can be implemented in workplaces. How do practitioners keep up to date; how can they evaluate what is useful and applicable research? This is precisely the area that need exploring to progress in occupational health, safety and environment practice. The need to meld the scientific, medical and technological aspects of these topics with the legal and social scientific analyses is pressing and not yet achieved. Some hazards and related risks still do need to be identified – low level exposures and mixed exposures to physical, chemical and biological hazards or all three immediately spring to mind – and measured and their health effects understood. But there is little need to constantly replicate the same research across the world whereas there is a desperate need to work out effective interventions and to implement control measures that are well understood. For many workers and communities, this does not entail blue skies scientific research but rather basic research on how to roll out existing good practice sometimes requiring little money and little technology. HSE in the past have provided a few good examples of how to do this, for instance, in dealing with noise problems, but more examples are needed.

Worker knowledge and professional practice limits

Much current public health policy relates to the need to consult users and consumers and to draw on community concerns in the development of health plans that reflect those concerns. This may pose major problems for the public health professional in terms of both identifying the relevant and representative audience, contacting them and then acting upon the concerns identified that may differ from or possibly conflict with the analysis and concerns of the health professional.

The position in workplaces may be similar in some respects in that employee perceptions and concerns about hazards may not coincide with those of occupational health and safety staff. Risk perceptions and risk assessments differ greatly in certain circumstances between lay and professional groups: it is important to recognise that such differences are not necessarily indications of better or worse judgements (Watterson 1998). As Table 9.2 shows, sometimes lay assessments based on different types of knowledge to professionals may well identify and document workplace hazards

Table 9.2   Lay assessments of hazards based on different types of knowledge available

Investigator	Hazard	Action
Alfred Greenwood, Glass Bottle Maker Secretary 1891 using social insurance records	Cataracts in glass workers	1900s: compensation but no action on the process
Local woodworkers trade union Secretary observing workforce 1900s	Narcotic effects on African box through slowing heartbeat	Substitution with safer woods as best available local exhaust ventilation still created dust inhaled by workers
South Wales Dockers Union Secretary observed pitch dust exposure of briquette workers 1910–20	Skin cancer known for centuries in tar workers	1927 finally recognised as an industrial disease for briquette workers
Sheffield Occupational Health Project	Chrome ulceration	The project team found more cases in one Sheffield factory than were recorded for the nation in official records
Local unemployed centre in Sunderland	Mucous membrane disease in engineering workers	The centre revealed gross under-reporting of the disease

Source: Legge 1934; Watterson 1999.

and associated illnesses rather better than those of professionals for a variety of reasons. In practice, occupational health and safety professionals are wise to take workplace worries and observations seriously and to draw on the different types of knowledge and expertise that may exist on the shopfloor.

It may be less problematic for the occupational health and safety professionals to identify their user/consumer groups as they could have a captive audience or population: namely the workforce. Hence, the HSE identified good communications with employees as a major role for the health and safety professional. However, having a captive workforce does not ensure effective communications, informed consent and an empowered and active workforce

on health and safety matters. Trade unions and especially trade
union safety representatives provide an immediate and unique
route in to particular groups in ways that community health councils cannot although the Friends of the Earth Environmental
Justice 'agents' may provide a similar route and source of community
information on pollution problems in communities. A larger problem emerges when workforces are not organised and it is unclear
that HSE or other bodies have yet found effective means to ensure
that employees in non-unionised workplaces are always properly
informed and involved in workplace health and safety matters.
Where outworkers and homeworkers exist, this will be another
challenge and the question of SMEs and their employees is one
that is uppermost in HSE and professional body minds but with no
clear solution on communication, involvement of employees and
effective workplace health and safety actions yet established.

Effective public health action on occupational ill-health and accidents

Putting these approaches into practice is problematic and will
come from activity at different levels. Within the public health
plans in England, Wales and Scotland, there are references to the
influence of work on health and the need to address occupational
health and safety problems. There are also references to involving
the public in the development of public health strategies. Short-
term interventions such as HAZ have in some instances identified
occupational health as an issue. Primary Care Trusts have a role in
preparing 'local' health plans and these should include occupational ill-health and accidents at work as one area for action
perhaps linked to other initiatives within the HSE and health education bodies. There are occupational health and safety initiatives
in the various national health promotion bodies. For the occupational health and safety practitioner, it is important to link up with
the health promotion agenda and to influence it. For too long,
health promotion in the workplace has been focused on diet, exercise and smoking and has rarely related effectively to a need to
address work-caused and work-related ill-health. Bringing the two
elements together and ensuring effective action on both rather
than one to the exclusion of the other is needed. This will also

help deal with the victim-blaming and 'lifestyle' preoccupation critique of much health promotion and provide much needed workplace credibility to health promotion.

Some mechanisms and measures that may help to achieve this should come through the following interventions.

1. Greater accountability of employers and government through upstream pressures from the public, employees and what might be termed conventional means. In this context occupational health professionals may work through their professional organisations, through representation on government and industry committees and through lobbying and campaigning. Corporate manslaughter for instance would help to ensure far greater accountability of boards of directors and would raise awareness of senior managers as to the seriousness of their workplace actions. At the same time it would ensure that HSE Inspectors had a very powerful stick as well as persuasion carrots to use in their work.

2. Democratic control of services. This raises the issue of health and safety professionals increasing the impact of their practice through the adoption of an advocacy or facilitating role in their work. If occupational health and safety services were more accountable to users and communities, stronger actions and more preventative action might emerge. This is linked in with better governance and good ethical practices, greater community, 'consumer' and user input into services that are integral to good public health practice.

3. Sustainability of interventions linking occupational and environmental health. Again some practitioners have been anxious to ensure that work environment problems are linked to wider environmental problems. From the public health perspective, what happens in the workplace in terms of pollution control will impact upon those outside. This may be important in assessing workplace exposure and may be important in terms of specific community exposures. For instance, workers may be exposed to fume and dust hazards in the workplace and, as often happens especially in developing countries, they may be exposed to the same hazards from the same sources when they leave work and go to their homes near workplaces and industrial complexes. They may additionally be exposed

to the same or similar contaminants through soil, water and food contamination. This is a form of what may be quadruple or even greater jeopardy. The occupational health and safety practitioner, with engineers, will be in a pivotal position to work on cutting both the workplace pollution and the wide pollution through strategies such as toxics-use reduction and sunsetting dangerous materials.

A number of these issues are also addressed in the chapter dealing with environmental health. Social justice and equity of resource distribution and means to address the uneven distribution of hazards between socio-economic groups. Practitioners can rarely deal directly with such problems and must rely on government policy, the law and professional institution lobbying. Statistical data within the United Kingdom and beyond quickly identify the most hazardous and unhealthy industries and occupations and often these recruit from the most vulnerable and lowest paid workers in those societies. Within hazardous industries and companies, all too often the lower the socio-economic position of the employee, the more hazardous the work will be and the greater the risk will be. Occasionally, occupational stress and repetitive strain injuries break that pattern but rarely.

One recent development that health and safety practitioners should be wary of is the tendency of some epidemiological studies not simply to adjust for socio-economic factors but to try and explain away any occupational or environmental health problems using the Carstairs index on deprivation. Those with the greatest workplace hazards usually face the greater immediate pollution and environmental hazards, for instance, in terms of siting of chemical plants, disposal of wastes, location of incinerators. These are central concerns of environmental and workplace justice measures to ensure that workers are not discriminated against either overtly or covertly on the grounds of ethnicity and gender. Black and migrant workers are disproportionately found in the most dangerous and unhealthy jobs (Watterson 1999). Lack of research has also occurred on hazards relating to gender: for instance work on occupational causes of breast cancer. Women also face more work-related upper limb disorders (WRULDS), violence and stress at work in traditional female occupations (www.hazards.org/women). Part-time/temporary workers also need better protection as there are 2.7 million non-permanent contracts. It is unclear currently how health and safety professionals will deal with these very specific challenges.

As with other public health professionals, occupational health and safety practitioners should be advocates and champions of their disciplines and the populations that they represent (Box 9.3). Prevention of occupational diseases and accidents is the primary task and this may be achieved by better occupational health services that pick up health problems earlier and document them more accurately and fully. Such data are needed to inform effective preventive measures and to pick up hazards that have slipped through the net or been underestimated. Many UK workers lack access to occupational health services. The NHS failed in the past to provide effective occupational health services for its own employees and was not set up to reach employees in other workplaces.

Box 9.3   Possible practitioner solutions to occupational health and safety problems

Need for occupational health and safety practitioners at all levels and in all organisations – governmental, public and private sectors to pursue a leader rather than a follower role in tackling workplace hazards for instance by use of hazard identification/removal and precautionary principle strategies at a very early stage.

Better effective linkage between occupational health and safety and environmental professionals.

Pressure to increase resources and staff within organisations and at governmental level.

Pressure to ensure development of effective occupational health services such as the pioneering primary care occupational health project in Sheffield (SOHP) that span disciplines, use expertise within communities and are readily available. NHS Plus does not follow the innovative SOHP model and has yet to be evaluated as to its range and effectiveness.

Pooling resources to raise SME health and safety standards.

Pressing for HSE to implement and then extend revitalising health and safety targets and carry forward plans on social exclusion, environmental justice, and socio-economic influences on health and safety.

Use available resources in workforces and trade unions more fully to advance health and safety practice.

Adopt wider and more active advocacy roles not only at national but also at local and workplace levels.

The United Kingdom has failed in the past to meet the EU directive on providing non self-referral occupational health services for the nation's workforce and has failed to ratify the ILO Convention on occupational health. Also in recent years, access to occupational health services has declined in the United Kingdom and we do not yet know how successful NHS Plus and other similar initiatives will be in redressing the balance in 2002.

A practitioner's charter

Hazard and risk control and their distribution depend on the economy, social structure and resources of a country as well as technical skills and knowledge. The following measures would ensure more effective interventions by the practitioner and assist in the search for best practice or good practice and not simple compliance with minimum and sometimes poor legal standards.

• *Precautionary principles to underpin all occupational health and safety practice*   (Raffensperger *et al.* 1999). The burden of proof should lie with manufacturers of equipment, plant, substances and the developers of systems of work to prove their products and systems are healthy and safe and where possible, these are the data that practitioners should search for. This presents a major challenge for those societies, industries, companies and organisations where full costs and sometimes any costs of occupational diseases and accidents are not borne by the employer. For instance, asbestos-related illnesses have often been contested and have remained uncompensated for in a number of instances until the worker has died from the illness. If full costs are paid, such payments could make some companies and organisations bankrupt: in these settings it is economically as well as ethically and legally unacceptable to ignore effective and best practice health and safety action.

• *Development of participatory research approaches and funding based on* worker/community/lay epidemiology empowering workers and communities in the investigation of hazards along the lines of the WHO European Charter on Environment and Health. This ensures that employers draw on the skills and knowledge of employees to identify hazards and explore means to remove hazards. In this context the health and safety practitioner may be the facilitator of progress and the champion of change.

• Planning up stream focus bringing together programmes that reduce workplace hazard exposures, cut pollution, benefit local community health and ensure plants are economical in their use of resources, investors in the most efficient plant and profitable. These are win–win approaches for health and safety professionals to advocate. For example, toxics-use reduction, sunsetting of hazardous and unsafe processes and materials.

• Worker/community based occupational/environmental health centres to be established or expanded along the lines of successful models in Italy, Scandinavia, the United States and the United Kingdom. Such centre would have major roles in occupational disease prevention and their secondary roles would relate to disease and accident treatment. These centres would be multi-disciplinary in nature, including ergonomists, physiotherapists, psychologists and worker/community representatives. The services would therefore also be an important part of the democratisation of occupational health and ensure that the public health model of occupational health rather than the medical model – disease treatment, health screening, rehabilitation oriented model – dominated. These programmes would draw on 'best practice' identified by the Sheffield Occupational Health Project. Centres would have the ability to target workplace populations exposed to particular hazards: for instance chemical workers or construction workers.

• Regulation to underpin good occupational health and safety practice is needed with powerful incentives for organisations to comply with the law and some certainty that regular inspections and meaningful enforcement will assist compliance. Effective and effectively enforced legislation to protect workers from illnesses and accidents at work including substantial fines, suspension from rights to become directors and imprisonment for serious offenders. 'Tough on the causes of occupational ill-health, tough on criminal employers who damage or threaten health and safety of employees.'

• This will require an adequately staffed, adequately funded HSE that can build on its useful role with regard to information and advice about how to deal with hazards and its very limited and for some ineffective enforcement role. HSE/HSC can develop further their good practice and advocacy roles to the benefit of occupational health and safety professionals.

- Health and safety professionals need to be able to influence supra-national organisations. An effective EU health and safety structure and proper support from within the United Kingdom for EU, ILO and WHO policies, is needed to improve worker health capable of preventing bodies such as the World Trade Organisation (WTO) sanctioning schemes which damage the health of workers and the communities in which they live.
- Effective and properly resourced freedom of information measures for those working in health and safety is critical to ensure that problems can be identified and action taken. Numerous reports in the United Kingdom, Australia and the United States produced by governments, economists and academics have shown that poor health and safety is a major financial burden for any society. Cutting ill-health at work is therefore a cost-effective measure. To save money, make workplaces more efficient, productive and environmentally safe, we need better occupational health standards, practices and services in the United Kingdom.

References

Abrams HK (2001) A short history of occupational health. *J Public Health Policy* **22**(1): 34–80.

Castleman B (1996) *Asbestos: Medical and Legal Aspects*, 4th edn. Aspen Law and Business, Frederick, Maryland.

DETR (2001) Revitalising Health and Safety: strategy document. DETR, London.

European Centre for Occupational Health, Safety and the Environment (ECOHSE) (www.gla.ac.uk/ecohse).

European Environment Agency (2001) *Late Lessons from Early Warnings: The Precautionary Principle 1896–2000*. EEA, Copenhagen.

Greene G (1971) *It's a Battlefield*. Penguin, Harmondsworth.

Hazards (1999) Issue 65: 1–2.

Hazards (2000) Issue 70: 14–15.

Hazards (2000) Issue 71: 13.

HSE (2001a) *The Costs to Britain of Workplace Accidents and Work Related Ill Health in 1995/6*. HSE, London.

HSE (2001b) *Health and Safety Statistics 2000/01*. HMSO, London.

IOSH (2001) *Professionals in Partnership*. IOSH, Leicester.

LaDou J (ed.) (1997) *Occupational and Environmental Medicine*, 2nd rev. edn. Appleton Lange, California.

Ladou J *et al.* (2001) International Code of Conduct (Ethics) for Occupational Health and Safety Professionals. *IJOEH* **7**(3): 230–2.

Legge T (1934) *Industrial Maladies*. Oxford University Press, Oxford.

OHAC (2002) *Report and Recommendations on Improving Access to Occupational Health Support*. HSC, London.

O'Neill R (2002) When it comes to health and safety, your life should be in union hands. *ILO Labour Education* **126**: 13–18.

Peto J, Decarli A, Vecchia C, Levi F and Negri E (1999) The European mesothelioma epidemic. *Br J Cancer* **79**(3): 666–72.

Raffensperger C and Tickner J (1999) *Protecting the Public Health and the Environment: Implementing the Precautionary Principle*. Island Press, Washington DC.

Takala J (1999) *Introductory Report of the ILO on Occupational Health and Safety*. ILO, Geneva.

Tudor O (2001) Grave concern: asbestos deaths. *Hazards* **74**: 4–5.

Tweedale G (1999) *Magic Mineral to Killer Dust: Turner and Newall and the Asbestos Hazard*. Oxford University Press, Oxford.

Watterson AE and Wright L (1998) *The Role of the Health and Safety Manager*, 2nd edn. Financial Times Management, London.

Watterson A (1998) 'Toxicology in the working environment' in Rose J (ed.) *Environmental Toxicology: Current Developments*. Gordon and Breach Science Publishers, Amsterdam, pp 225–52.

Watterson AE (1999) 'Why we still have "old" epidemics and "endemics" in occupational health' in Daykin N and Doyal L (eds) *Health and Work: Critical Perspective*. Macmillan, Basingstoke, pp 107–26.

Watterson A (2001) Agricultural science and food policy for consumers and workers: recipes for public health successes or disaster. *New Solutions* **10**(4): 317–24.

WHO (1996) *Global Strategy on Occupational Health for All*. WHO, Geneva.

WHO (1997) *Health and Environment in Sustainable Development*. WHO, Geneva.

Woolfson C, Foster J and Beck M (1996) *Paying for the Piper: Capital and Labour in Britain's Offshore Oil Industry*. Mansell, London.

10

Health Promotion and the Role of the Health Promotion Specialist

Steve Bell

Introduction

Many people and many resources are devoted globally to 'health promotion'. Yet, health promotion is plagued critically by four major problems. The first problem is almost unique to this field. The last three problems are common to many public health professionals. They are:

- a confused identity
- political baggage
- a firm evidence base
- dependence on others.

This chapter will explore the work of health promotion specialist staff focusing on a regional UK health body. It will examine the tensions, conflicts, challenges and opportunities experienced by health promoters in their work and illustrate these elements through a number of small case studies. Such activity is underpinned by the health promotion philosophy described below, by the policy demands and expectations of national and regional bodies, by professional standards and good practice, by resources and staffing at a strategic, tactical *and functional* level and by such issues as catalytic leadership, team composition, team working, handling conflicts, building partnerships, training, facilitating, communicating and sometimes *social* marketing campaigns. There are technical as well as purely 'management' challenges and often they come together. On what basis are budgets allocated: for instance, who determines budgets on audio–visual aids and pamphlet expenditure and why? Who evaluates this material? What is the balance between information provision and policy/advocacy/ networking work?

The way that health promotion departments relate to public health medicine, primary care and community nursing are discussed in Chapters 3 and 4 and some different perspectives on the nature and practice of health promotion are offered there? Does the relationship change when health promotion departments operate under the same umbrella as these generic public health or medical and nursing teams as opposed to when they operate independently? If so, how does the relationship change? How are common issues and campaigns decided upon and actioned? How are public health and health promotion strategies and tactics decided upon? A number of these questions are dealt with in this chapter. Addressing such challenges requires appropriate skills and resources for appropriate groups and linked to a holistic view of health promotion (Allegrante *et al.* 2001; Holdke 2001; Long and Baxter 2001).

What is health promotion?

Health promotion draws on the World Health Organisation (WHO) view of upstream and downstream public health with health promotion located increasingly as an upstream activity. The health promotion movement has been described as 'a radical one which challenges the medicalisation of health, stresses its social and economic aspects, and portrays health as having a central place in a flourishing human life' (Downie *et al.* 1990: 1). The same commentators define health promotion as the 'efforts to enhance positive health and prevent ill-health, through the overlapping spheres of health education, prevention and health protection' (Downie *et al.* 1990: 2). This would suggest that health promotion is complex, diverse, multi-faceted and challenging to health promoters themselves, politicians, the medical profession and the public and that the 'discipline' needs to be responsive and reflective in its practice.

A search of entries appearing under the subject title of health promotion on the British Library database produces a rich and varied array of publications ranging from general textbooks through policy documents to those with a specific practice based focus. Perhaps the most interesting thing about the approximately 1000 items that appear is, however, that none predate 1979. Also, for some commentators 'health promotion' *per se* does not exist as a discrete entity and is absorbed within other policy and practice areas. For instance Beaglehole and Bonita in their review of public health do not provide one index reference to health promotion (Beaglehole and Bonita 1997). In the mid-1990s, UK Chief Medical Officer Annual Reports on the state of the public health would often include subjects that related to health promotion interventions yet health promotion as a strategy and method was sometimes not highlighted at all or marginalised in references to workplace health promotion activity (Department of Health 1995: iii–vii). The struggle for credibility of the discipline among medical staff has been a long one although in 2002, health promotion is firmly located within public health departments.

The roots of health promotion lay in what went before. Health promotion history is as long as the bio-medical tradition to which it is often regarded as a counterpoint and is identifiable in the deep antiquity of classical Greek and Minoan civilisations. What we would today recognise as health promotion emerged more recently as a construct of the post-modern condition from a melting pot of health education, anti-authoritarianism, anti-globalisation, the green and women's movement, chaos theory and the diminishing returns of the bio-mechanical medical model. Coming to occupy ground already occupied by the New Public Health, health promotion represented a rediscovery of the Victorian public health movement, and emerged into a relative void.

The politics of health promotion

For a subject area so new, it has risen quickly up the political and media agendas perhaps because the activity will always lie somewhere along the spectrum of libertarianism and authoritarianism; a spectrum that arouses powerful political and public passions. Achieving consensus about the importance of health promotion is, however, somewhat more straightforward than achieving consensus about what the term means and represents, and despite many attempts to introduce definitions. In essence, the problem is that the term health promotion is used to describe many different things, and even more problematically, all may be right. These may include:

- Political constructs of health promotion that focus on the relationship of power and the individual, and the inalienable right to equity in power and in health, such as that championed by the Health For All movement.
- Functional definitions that see health promotion characterised as a range of methodologies and approaches, such as that proposed by Fyfe, Tannahill and Tannahill.
- Functional constructs that represent health promotion as features of organisations, such as health promotion departments, and most problematically for health promotion specialists, functional descriptions in relation to a specific occupational group.
- Tactical definitions which see health promotion as a process which is characterised by a set of levers.

So what may be 'distinctive about health promotion is the attention that it gives to the facilitation of healthy lives: the idea that it is no good just telling people that they should change their lifestyles without also altering their social, economic and ecological environments. People must be able to live healthy lives. Health promotion aims to work not only at the level of individuals but also at the level of socio-economic structures and to encourage the creation and implementation of "healthy public policies" such as those concerned with transport, environment, agriculture and so on' (Bunton *et al.* 1995: 2).

The World Health Organisation Ottawa Charter (1986), defines five key levers which may enable people to take control over and improve their health. These are through:

- building healthful public policy
- creating supportive environments
- strengthening Community Action
- developing personal skills
- reorienting health services.

There are other views of health promotion. Three widely held views among the public and some health professionals are first that 'health promotion' can be done by everyone and so requires no special expertise or group; second that the subject is simply 'common sense' although common sense is rarely defined; and third that the subject is an unnecessary intrusion into individual freedom. Some have important reservations about the health and illness statistics base that can skew medical and health promotion interventions. For example 'when women's health problems are identified in health promotion, these tend to be medicalised leading at times to inappropriate and ineffective solutions. In addition health promotion strategies may place responsibility for health on women without recognising their relative lack of power to effect change. The victim-blaming that results from conventional health promotion approaches impacts upon women as carers, by ignoring the socio-economic context and social marginalisation of that caring role' (Daykin and Naidoo 1995: 59). Health promotion campaigns on passive smoking, alcohol consumption and accidents to children could all produce victim-blaming of women if the wider social, political and economic root causes of these health problems were not identified and addressed.

Among health promoters there may also be views about their role as advocates of public health which could then simply lead to empowering communities and the built-in self-destruction of the profession. It is unlikely that such empowerment will emerge either widely or quickly.

Who are health promoters?

Health promotion specialists are perhaps best characterised in terms of their diversity, and it is within this diversity that both their strength and, ironically, weaknesses are to be found. In the United Kingdom, health promoters may come from an NHS background, frequently in Nursing, Dietetics and Professions Allied to Medicine. Health promotion specialists are almost unique within the health service in that as a group, many of their numbers have origins external to the NHS. The skills and experiences derived from time spent as, for instance, teachers, social workers and community activists, bring a richness to health promotion and the wider NHS, and perhaps underpin the strength of health promotion to transcend traditional barriers and engage in effective partnership working. Health promotion specialists will also work closely with and possibly in the same organisation as public health physicians and nurses, pharmacists, dentists, teachers and social service staff, Professions Allied to Medicine, the police, primary care health professionals, psychiatrists, community psychiatric nurses, mental health staff, policy analysts and so on. Box 10.1 produced by Finnie and Nicolson illustrates in some detail how for instance focused clinical interventions by nurses might have health promotion benefits for those marginalised and most vulnerable in the community.

Box 10.1   Promoting health at a wound care clinic for
homeless people – a multi-layered approach to
a multi-layered clinical problem

Drug abuse is increasing globally, and has huge implications for health care practitioners. Together with rising numbers of injecting drug users, there are associated physical and mental health implications, many drug users experience feelings of low self worth, paranoia, anxiety and depression.

Homeless people are four times more likely to misuse drugs. They already have problems in nearly every aspect of daily living, from having somewhere to stay, to accessing nutritious food, accessing money, keeping clothes clean, to just staying warm. Each day is a potential struggle, and combined with drug addiction and the associated physical and mental health difficulties, homeless people may struggle to care for themselves, and many also have difficulties accessing health services (Scottish Executive, 2000).

The problem of access extends to many areas of healthcare in the NHS, but most commonly in GP practices and Accident and Emergency

Departments. Reports of being treated like social lepers by medical and nursing staff are commonplace in homeless and drug services. Lack of appropriate training, combined with irrational prejudice, largely cultivated by the media, leads to a breakdown in practitioner–client relationships that can be irreparable. Significantly, health promotion opportunities are not only being missed by health practitioners, but spectacularly damaged. Appropriate engagement with homeless people and drug users can open up excellent opportunities to promote the well-being of an individual and lay the foundation for future appointments being non-confrontational, constructive and therapeutic.

Drug misuse is a complex problem and an individual may fare better if given an opportunity to address the problem with support from a drugs worker: this is an illness avoidance and health promotion opportunity. If Methadone is offered as part of the treatment, the individual is likely to try to stop or reduce drug-related activities, which previously took up most of their day. Users need something to replace this, therefore support packages and alternatives to a drug-using lifestyle must be explored. Sometimes drug-users on Methadone are still injecting, as it can take some time for people to achieve stability in their drug use. Unfortunately some drug services and GP's give absolutely no leeway for drug users to make mistakes, and will withdraw Methadone prescriptions if a patient is thought to be continuing to inject or use other illegal substances. The drug-user may therefore hide drug use and also hide resultant health complications from risk-taking behaviour. This will range from HIV and hepatitis exposure to concealment of abscesses and ulcers through injecting.

Skin care is often a low priority for drug using individuals but is a frequent cause of morbidity in the homeless population. In a survey conducted by the Big Issue in the North (1998) of Big Issue Magazine Vendors a variety of health problems were identified. 26% of those surveyed identified skin problems compared to the General Household survey where people reported only a 1% incidence of skin disease. The Royal College of Physicians (RCP) report in 1994 found that 24% of homeless people had skin and persistent foot trouble – citing examples of leg ulcers, head lice and scabies (RCP 1994). Not all of these are chronic problems, but some are serious and early identification of infection can be life-saving. Those with skin problems may as a last resort attend Accident and Emergency Departments rather than wound care clinics or GP practices, and generally may be reluctant to attend any 'authoritarian' venue for care.

As a result, they may look out with mainstream health care for advice and treatment. The Big Issue in Scotland has set up a health project that endeavours to be flexible, easy to access, friendly and attractive to homeless people. This comprises services such as nursing, chiropody, physiotherapy, dental, hairdressing and complementary therapies; and in addition a wound care clinic. Assessment of skin problems is undertaken and treatment offered where appropriate. Skin disease may be a result of injecting behaviour, the quality, solvency, and cleanliness of the drug, the equipment and the environment. Long-term injecting drug-use can result in sclerosis and thrombosis of most superficial veins and if venous access is no longer possible users may resort to skin or muscle popping, where injecting occurs directly through the skin surface and the drug is absorbed subcutaneously or from muscle. Women have a greater tendency to inject into muscle as a consequence of poor venous access. This approach can result in abscess formation, and infection and frequent scarring may result with multiple circular scars (Finnie and Nicolson 2002). The Big Issue venue is viewed as a 'safe' and neutral area but alcohol and drugs are not permitted on the premises. Many individuals with skin problems use the opportunity to chat about other aspects of their lives and in this informal setting health promotion opportunities may be available. General discussion may involve areas such as nutrition, alcohol and drug use, safe injecting practices, housing, relationships – in fact, anything that may impact on a drug-users lifestyle, and subsequently their health. There is a lack of evidence for the management of physical health in this population and equally the impact of health promotion advice in this group has not been evaluated, however compliance and regular attendance by users has been achieved possibly through promoting an equal and accessible service which is non-judgemental or authoritarian. The service has been welcomed by users who appreciate easy access to health care professionals.

Alison Finnie, Department of Nursing and Midwifery, University of Stirling and Paul Nicolson, Manager, Health Project' Big Issue Foundation, Scotland

Reference List

The Big Issue in the North Trust (1998) A Primary Healthcare Study of Vendors of The Big Issue in The North. The Big Issue in The North Trust, Manchester.

Finnie, A. and Nicolson, P. (2002) Injecting drug use and implications for skin and wound management. *British Journal of Nursing* (Supplement) **11**, 6.

Royal College of Physicians (1994) Homelessness and Ill Health. London: Royal College of Physicians.

Scottish Executive (2000) Report of the Glasgow Street Homelessness Review Team. Edinburgh: Scottish Executive.

A key distinction therefore needs to be made between the health promoter – into which category all of the above health professional groups should and typically do fall – with health promotion representing at least a part of their responsibilities; and the Health Promotion Specialist, who is characterised as such in the sense that health promotion comprises their entire *raison d'etre*.

Health promoters may be located in varied settings and use many techniques and methods in their work. They may for instance work for health departments, education departments, in primary care, government agencies and non-governmental organisations (NGOs). They may, for example, focus on delivering health promotion to the public, they may develop health promoting materials in a variety of media, they may pursue strategic goals and influence and advise key health professional staff, they may combine several of these tasks. Health promoting activities are not only varied but they may be complex and influenced in several different ways by international policy through WHO, by National Government strategy which in the United Kingdom would come through the Department of Health in England and the Scottish Executive Health Department. There may also be national professional guidelines, regional and local public health strategies and particular patient or community agendas. Health promotion may be developed, directed or thwarted by a range of factors – policy, practice, legal, financial and staffing.

In the United Kingdom, resources are relatively generous but there is a shortage of trained health promotion staff to carry out the work: this can have a significant impact on the effectiveness of health promotion programmes and health promotion groups.

Circumstances will vary as to particular facilitating factors or barriers (von dem Knesebeck *et al.* 2001). Methods and philosophies of health promotion may be similar but target groups or locations may differ enormously and hence necessitate the design of specific programmes. For instance, health promotion programmes as a means to prevent HIV in sex workers in South Africa had to take account of how 'community dynamics have shaped the peer education programme's development in a deprived, violent community where existing norms and networks are inconsistent with ideal criteria for participatory health promotion' (Campbell *et al.* 2001, 1978). Peer education programmes have been used in Leicestershire to reach Asian communities in an effort to reduce risk factors for coronary heart diseases because primary care teams had previously been unable to influence developments. The programme helped to change GP attitudes and provided substantial lay education on the subject (Farooqi and Bhavsar 2001). The impact on the coronary heart disease figures will of course not be known for some considerable time assuming it is possible to tease out the specific influence of this health promotion programme on those figures. Populations too will differ in terms of disease profiles. For instance, health promoters would often view socially deprived inner city areas as most likely to demonstrate serious and extensive heart disease problems across a large population. Rural and remote areas would be viewed as problematic because of access. However, rural Manitoba in Canada has the highest cardiovascular disease risk factors and the lowest level of heart-related knowledge when compared with urban areas in the same province. This led to 'rural community committee-driven approach with appropriate training, limited resources and at a low cost' to address the health promotion problem identified (Harvey *et al.* 2001: 31).

Role of health promotion departments

These may vary in a number of respects related to their location, funding and staffing as well as their overall philosophy and practice of the espoused philosophy. Chapter 3 located health promotion within the context of public health departments and provides a quite detailed insight into how the health promotion team defined in very broad terms addresses such issues as food and nutrition. Chapter 4 provides an assessment of 'forced health promotion' in primary care where GPs were rewarded for introducing certain initiatives whether they were 'needed', evaluated or not. Such forcing led to a range of positive initiatives, some failed initiatives and much scepticism generated by GPs in the process about the effectiveness of the whole discipline. This section looks at organically generated and valued health promotion departments.

Health promotion departments for instance in Scotland are attached to Scottish NHS Boards, some being with the Board itself, typically within Public Health Directorates, with some being within Primary Care Trusts. There is presently some debate about the most appropriate location and orientation of health promotion. Roles and functions are relatively similar, though scale does vary significantly from one to another. In the Highlands, the Health Promotion Department comprises one manager, five lead health promotion staff, and a number of staff with a more project orientation (Box 10.2).

Broadly speaking, a Health Promotion Department located and configured in this way has four main functions.

- Ensuring the provision of specialist health promotion input at strategic, policy and functional levels, both regionally and locally.
- Adding value to the regional health promotion capacity through national liaison and resource accumulation.
- Managing and supporting specific regional programmes of work.
- Maintaining and developing the NHS Health Information and resources services in the region.

Box 10.2   A 'typical' health promotion team of 34 for an estimated 275 926 people in a mixed area of towns, cities and villages, industrial and rural activities with six public health physicians. The team comprises:

1 Health promotion manager
2 Office/clerical support staff
1 Community health promoter
1 Domestic violence worker
1 Health promoter in education
1 Health promotion support worker in education
3 Information and resource specialists
1 Oral and dental health promotion officer
1 Physical activity and accidents health promotion officer
4 Primary care health promoters and support workers
6 Sexual health promotion and support officers
1 Smoking cessation officer
2 Substance use health promoters
3 Workplace health promoters and support workers
6 Nutrition and dietetics staff with 1 secretary

Forth Valley Health Board. 11th Annual Health Report on Public Health 1999/2000 (Stirling 2000).

Who are health promotion specialists?

As indicated earlier, the entry route for health promotion specialists is wide and varied, and the reasons for entering the field is similarly diverse. Historically, a career as a health promotion specialist was viewed, particularly, by those in teaching and nursing, as a 'promoted post' in the sense of having a wider scope and the potential of impacting at a tactical and strategic level, if not also in terms of remuneration. This wider sense of scope, and the genuine feeling of frustration of 'pulling the bodies from the river' is another reason for wishing to become engaged; many people working in health promotion would also cite a strong ethical and even political motivation, for health promotion is ultimately a political act. It is concerned with empowerment which, demystifying the jargon, is about redistributing power from one group to another. In its extreme, health promotion could even be characterised as a crusade, indeed it is often this element that generates most criticism, frequently drawing the jibe of 'health police'.

What do health promoters do?

Their tasks may be many and varied. Internationally, the agenda for health has been set by the WHO and during recent decades, it has promulgated Health For All targets for different regions of the world that have been taken up by various national governments and agencies. There have also been WHO programmes on Healthy Cities, Healthy Schools, Healthy Hospitals and Healthy Communities that functioned in different ways in different countries (Stanton *et al.* 1996; Deccache *et al.* 2001; Aujoulat *et al.* 2001). These programmes in the United Kingdom were often used as a means of circumventing less than supportive national governments, such as the Thatcher Administration of the 1980s which attempted to bury the Black Report on health inequalities and also to stifle important health initiatives. These WHO programmes have influenced health promoters and provided a framework for action and a set of targets to move public health policy towards. In the United Kingdom health promotion has had a major role to play in the Health of the Nation and Our Healthier Nation strategies.

Most English, Welsh and Scottish health plans now contain programmes that deal with life circumstances and inequalities, lifestyles, prevention of ill-health and treatment and care. The first three categories entail major input from health promoters and usually operate together with interventions and programmes that operate at different levels.

The health promotion experience in the Highlands of Scotland

This is 'knitted' into a coherent public health strategy that looks at individual, community and national activity and includes the recognition that public health and health promotion entails 'fiscal, political and policy' changes (Highland Health Board 2001: 5).

An integral part of the strategy revolves around 'partnership working' and these partnerships involve health promoting activities. For instance, the Highland Wellbeing Alliance brings together the Highland Health Board, the council, the Enterprise Board, the police, Housing, environmental and voluntary groups. To promote healthy and safe and sustainable communities, a health promotion strategy and input is needed. Health promotion contributes to the generation and circulation of information about domestic abuse and hence raising awareness.

The information and communication role of health promotion for health professionals and communities should not therefore be underestimated but its major role has historically been in the area of 'lifestyles'. Even here, there have been significant UK-wide developments with an emphasis more on developing policies and frameworks within which individuals will be able and empowered to make choices. There will be strategic decisions for health promoters to take in terms of identifying particular and high threats to health in a region and resources, staff and the search for effectiveness will mean that it is impossible to have major initiatives on all health issues all of the time. Within the Highlands for instance, diet and nutrition, alcohol use and road accidents are particular concerns along with the national targets on coronary heart disease – linked to nutrition, cancer stroke, teenage pregnancies and smoking.

Case studies on lifestyle work of health promoters

The rights of communities to good health with regard to remedying social injustice, ensuring social inclusion and dealing with the impact of poverty are part of a health promoter's work on life circumstances. The key players in such activity will be policy makers and community leaders. The focus for action in health promotion often reflects national public health priorities and hence may be determined by regional assessments of those priorities. In this respect, health promotion activities of health boards, PCTs and PCGs are all important.

Within the life circumstances framework, there are lifestyle issues that relate more to individual responsibilities if the poverty and resource issues are addressed. Hence, access to good quality fresh fruit and vegetables for instance depends on removing physical, geographic and other barriers. Effective smoking cessation programmes will operate where there is proper support for those wishing to participate. This is where the health promotion specialist would work with other public health professionals to identify and plan effective interventions through a potentially large number of health, education and social services professionals out in community locations who could introduce or facilitate appropriate interventions and campaigns and work with the public on their success. In some instances, health promotion departments may target health professional groups such as nurses to increase the knowledge base and skills of those likely to be directly involved either in primary care or other health care sectors.

In the Highlands, the health board health promotion team plays a major part in the delivery of health promotion modules to student nurses. In the United States, researchers found that nursing students needed to have relevant health promotion integrated into student learning in order to ensure the subject had maximum impact on those students (Jacobson *et al.* 1998). There may also be some value in the design and delivery of bespoke health promotion programmes for specific groups such as those working in paediatrics (Kataoka-Yahiro *et al.* 2001). We may then be able to evaluate the effectiveness of such education on the nurses but what we do not yet know is how effective those nurses will be in promoting health and changing lifestyles of their patients. Recent research appears to indicate that despite an increase in health promotion and health education practice, 'nurses have been and continue to be ineffective and inconsistent health education practitioners' (Whitehead 2001: 417). Whitehead moots the solution of widely adopted social cognitive behavioural models of health promotion by nurses: how effective such a strategy would be in improving population health has again yet to be evaluated.

Efforts to address 'lifestyle' can be categorised into five principal areas:

- Removing physical barriers to access, such as the poor availability of fresh fruit and vegetables or unaffordable leisure opportunities.
- Ensuring that appropriate support is available for people wanting to change their lifestyle, such as smoking cessation support.
- Developing individual and community capacities, such as lifeskills, self-efficacy and self-esteem.
- Improving knowledge by providing accurate, consistent and accessible information.
- Creating a positive health culture, in which health is seen as a partnership effort in which we all have a stake.

Case study one: nutrition

The role of public health workers in nutrition runs the gamut of health to illness, public health interventions to clinical interventions, community to individuals. Health promoters could have a role upstream or downstream. Meredith Turshen, for instance, saw nutrition health promotion activity upstream coming from reorganised land reform, organic farming, pesticide-use reduction strategies, use of appropriate technologies, varied seed stock and good credit arrangements. Downstream interventions would mean a focus on nutrition education, vitamin supplement campaigns, supplementary feeding programmes such as school lunches, breakfast clubs and fresh fruit provision (Turshen 1989: 188–201). In other settings health promoters especially in the United States have viewed their work as advocates/upstream interventionists by bussing community members in deprived areas to those supermarkets that did not raise prices when benefit cheques were due. These activities all relate to removing physical barriers to access.

The shift of opinion on food subjects has in some instances been surprising with public health physicians looking upstream and voicing opinions about, for instance, the need to adopt the precautionary principle and oppose genetic crop experimental trials in Scottish regions like Lothian. In the mainstream, health promoters are attempting to engage with food producers and retailers to increase access to fruits and vegetables. Community nutrition assistants are likewise a possible option to take forward such initiatives as Weaning Parties, Cook and Eat sessions and Food Co-ops. Efforts are being made too to influence the curriculum of catering courses and include healthy eating and healthy recipe module development. The challenge comes for health promoters to ensure that such initiatives receive core funding and are sustained after pilot interventions have been evaluated.

Case study two: sexual health

Sexual health including the reduction of unwanted teenage pregnancies are Highland health promotion priorities in the context of a holistic and positive approach. A range of interventions have been developed. These include programmes to address low confidence and esteem in young people through assertiveness training with pupils in community schools, through training and updating of key professional staff especially by reaching key education and school nurse staff.

To break down concerns that young people may have about the stigma of sexual diseases and the threat to confidentiality which they may perceive, the 'Walk the Talk' initiative was devised. This provides training and support to primary care staff such as nurse and doctors and also receptionists to ensure there are youth friendly medical practices in the area. At the same time, a Highland-wide Youth Advice Service accessible by phone and e-mail has been developed to lessen concerns about personal embarrassing direct face-to-face approaches with health workers and to address equity issues of those young people in rural and remote areas who would not have access to services directly anyway. This has been linked to additional work with young people on confidentiality and young people's rights and research programmes to reach previously excluded groups especially young people from ethnic minority backgrounds.

Case study three: injecting drug misuse

Health promoters have worked in the substance use field over many decades. In recent years Highland partnership working through the Highland Drug and Alcohol Strategy Group has been a major plank in taking forward health promotion policies based on evidence provided by researchers on the type, extent and distribution of drug use in the region and data on the harm done. Pharmacists and needle exchanges helped provide clean needles but nevertheless 46 per cent of a survey sample of 76 injecting drug users had still shared a needle in the last six months and 84 per cent of the same sample had had sexual intercourse with a member of the opposite sex in that same period. Following the research findings, the health promotion team worked on ensuring more information reached the users with regard to injection risks and sexual disease risks, improving needle and syringe exchange facilities in the region, making drug user services more relevant, user friendly and accessible and implementing a hepatitis B immunisation programme for injecting drug users. This provides some interesting similarities and contrasts with the Finnie and Nicolson case study cited earlier.

The evidence base for health promotion

The lack of an evidence base for many medical and health promotion interventions means that it is difficult to establish what impact downstream interventions may have although they will often be quite critical for individuals, families and communities. There has been much concern over decades primarily to ensure that health promotion interventions are evaluated to make sure they work, to ensure resources are not wasted and to improve approaches used (Downie *et al.* 1990: 73–4). Geoffrey Rose identified the prevention paradox in 1981 whereby 'a preventive measure that brings large benefits to the community offers little to each participating individual' (Rose 1992: 12). The effectiveness of health promotion interventions therefore need to be epidemiologically informed and presented in a public health rather than individual health context although health promoters themselves may well need to present individuals with clear if less significant benefits to be gained from particular health promotion campaigns.

Evidence about what impacts health promoters have had on producers and retailers to offer, encourage and maintain healthier diets through healthier foods purchases by their customers will be needed. Similar choices exist for health promoters in terms of tobacco. Working downstream with those addicted to help individuals stop smoking or to reduce exposures of young children to passive smoking is very important at the individual and family level. Taxing tobacco and preventing tobacco advertising requires national intervention and would be a role for a national group of health promoters as would be support for suggestions mooted within the WHO to make tobacco a 'prescription only' drug thereby recognising its addictive nature.

Health policy researchers have found that decision-makers may use evidence presented to them in both direct and indirect ways (Elliott and Popay 2000). The evaluation of health promotion impacts on the public is far more difficult to assess and may be quite indirect. The search for evidence of effective health promotion has been a long and tortuous one. In some respects, if access to information and the opportunity to empower individual health choices are achieved, the health promotion has met a key criterion for its existence and the activity demonstrates purpose even if outcomes cannot be demonstrated. This does not of course necessarily reflect value for money or evidence-based health practice. Researchers and practitioners have therefore been active in searching for tools to carry out the effectiveness assessment (Spellar *et al.* 1997: 361). To do this, Spellar and her colleagues consider they need assessments of a broader range of activities undertaken; systematic reviews that include a wider range of research methods especially qualitative research; and review criteria that looks at the 'quality of the…intervention as well as the research design' to ensure that poor quality interventions are not included in systematic reviews (Spellar *et al.* 1997: 362).

Conclusions

Health promoters have a role to play in the building of comprehensive and effective public health policies and practices. Such policies are contested for instances by the tobacco industry, the pharmaceutical industry and the alcohol industry, by advertisers and by lobbyists inimical to health objectives. Health promoters in NGOs, health promotion academics and those working through national professional groups may be able to press for such policies through effective practice. Health promoters at regional and local level can create environments that support their work and can link that work in with local government, health authority, education initiatives and partnership networks as well as with voluntary organisations and industry. Health promoters too can build up social capital and community strength to address some of the policy questions in ways the health promoters themselves may not be able to do directly. This may be achieved partly by building up personal, family, group and community skills and it could be done in the home, in playgroups and schools, workplace and hospitals, clinics and community centres, street corners and youth clubs, shops and leisure centres.

In the United Kingdom, there have historically been problems with the dominance of acute hospital services over both primary care and public health. It had long been the case that 'health care services, in their organisation and main theories of operation, do not support the promotion of good health' (Ashton and Seymour 1988: 84). Paradoxically hospitals have also had a very poor record in looking after the health of their own employees and the WHO Healthy Hospitals programme was designed to address some of these shortcomings. With the current UK emphasis on acute hospital services and, in England if not in Scotland, a crisis in primary care with the bureaucratisation and pharmaceutical indebtedness of PCTs, it may be a major challenge for some health promotion professionals to retain not just staff and funds but also practice at the interface between health sciences and social, economic, political and educational policy.

References

Allegrante JP, Moon RW, Auld ME and Gebbie KM (2001) Continuing education needs of the currently employed public health education workforce. *Am J Public Health* **91**(8): 2130–4.
Ashton J and Seymour H (1988) *The New Public Health*. Open University Press, Milton Keynes.

Aujoulat I, le Faou AL, Sandrin-Berthon B, Martin F and Deccache A (2001) Implementing health promotion in health care settings: conceptual coherence and policy support. *Patient Educ Couns* **45**(4): 245–54.

Beaglehole R and Bonita R (1997) *Public Health at the Crossroads.* Cambridge University Press, Cambridge.

Bunton R, Nettleton S and Burrows R (eds) (1995) *The Sociology of Health Promotion: Critical Analyses of Consumption, Lifestyle and Risk.* Routledge, London.

Campbell C and Mzaidume Z (2001) Grassroots participation, peer education and HIV prevention by sex workers in South Africa. *Am J Public Health* **91**(12): 1978–86.

Daykin N and Naidoo J (1995) 'Feminist critiques of health promotion' in Bunton *et al.* (eds) *The Sociology of Health Promotion: Critical Analyses of Consumption, Lifestyle and Risk.* Routledge, London, pp 60–9.

Deccache A and van Ballenkon K (2001) Patient education in Belgium: evolution, policy and perspectives. *Patient Educ Couns* **44**(1): 43–8.

Department of Health (1995) *On the State of the Public Health 1994.* HMSO, London.

Downie RS, Fyfe C and Tannahill A (1990) *Health Promotion: Models and Values.* Oxford University Press, Oxford.

Elliott H and Popay J (2000) How are policy makers using evidence? Models of research utilisation and local NHS policy making. *J Epidemiol Community Health* **54**: 461–8.

Farooqi A and Bhavsar M (2001) Project Dil: a co-ordinated primary care and community health promotion programme for reducing risk factors of coronary heart disease amongst the South Asian community of Leicester – experiences and evaluation of the project. *Eth Health* **6**(3–4): 265–70.

Harvey D, Hook E, McKay M, Cepanese D and Gelskey D (2001) Enhancement of rural community capacity for heart health promotion in Manitoba. *Promot Educ* (Suppl 1): 31–4.

Highland Health Board (2001) *Working Together for a Healthier Highland Annual Report of the Director of Public Health and Health Policy 2000–2001.* HHB, Inverness.

Holdke B (2001) New duties of the medical child health surveillance teams: the Hamburg Concept. *Gesundheitswesen* **63**(11): 672–6.

Jacobson SF, MacRobert M, Leon C and McKinnon E (1998) A faculty case management practice: integrated teaching, service and research. *Nurs Research Health care Perspect* **19**(5): 220–3.

Kataoka-Yahiro M, Tessier K, Ratcliffe C, Cohen J and Matsumoto-Oi D (2001) Learning-service community partnership model: a pediatric-program evaluation. *J Padiatric Nurs* **16**(6): 412–7.

Long A and Baxter R (2001) Functionalism and holism: community nurses' perceptions of health. *J Clin Nurs* **10**(3): 320–9.

Rose G (1992) *The Strategy of Preventive Medicine.* Oxford Medical Publications, Oxford.

Spellar V, Learmonth A and Harrison D (1997) The search for evidence of effective health promotion. *BMJ* **315**: 361–3.

Stanton WR, Balanda KP, Gillespie AM and Lowe JB (1996) Barriers to health promotion activities in public hospitals. *Aust NZ J Public Health* **20**(5): 500–4.

Turshen M (1989) *The Politics of Public Health.* Zed Books, London.

Von dem Knesbeck O, Badura B, Zamora P, Weihrauch B, Werse W and Siegrist J (2001) Evaluation of health policy interventions on the community level. *Gesundheitswesen* **63**(1): 35–41.

WHO and Health and Welfare Canada (1986) *The Ottowa Charter for Health Promotion.* WHO, Copenhagen.

Whitehead D (2001) A social cognitive model for health education/ health promotion practice. *J Adv Nurs* **36**(3): 417–25.

11

Conclusions

Andrew Watterson, Thomas Gorman,
James McCourt and Maureen Dennis

Public health practitioners operate with finite budgets and staff and struggle with maintaining, developing and applying technical skills to public health problems, adjusting to new challenges, addressing old problems and making sense of a plethora of political, economic, legal and organisational changes. How they do these things and move forward on a wide range of public health subjects has been described in some detail in the preceding chapters. They have moved from mono-professionalism towards multi-professionalism, individual and small team working to large team work and inter-disciplinary working. They have worked in geographically focussed specialist teams and have been dispersed to primary care bases. The numbers of 'dedicated' paid public health workers and their budgets have increased enormously in the last 150 years.

In the nineteenth century, many of the major challenges to public health were addressed by civil engineering, planning, housing, water supply and sanitary sciences with some important developments in biology, chemistry and microbiology. In some field, very limited scientific and medical knowledge led to major public health advances. In the twentieth century there was almost unbounded optimism about the capacity of science, medicine and related disciplines to ensure public health and extend the lifespan of any population. The practice of course only succeeded and then only partially in the northern hemisphere with wide differences in mortality and morbidity based on socio-economic differences. De facto global public health did not rank highly as a major concern in that hemisphere. Increasing the quality of life was not an objective for most governments, companies and international agencies at the time.

At the end of the twentieth century and the beginning of the twenty-first century, various analyses were offered on the beneficial impacts of 'globalisation' along with the recognition that the process 'threatens public health and the interests of poorer people in poorer countries' (Feacham 2002: 44, 2001). This was precisely at a time when the failures of global economic policies were being documented with serious effects on public health and welfare (Weisbrot *et al.* 2002; Horton 2001; Butler 2002). These failures occurred for instance on food security, water security, infectious diseases, global warming, maternal and child health. Also, the links between poor public health, poverty and poor primary care are close and the stronger the primary care is in a country, the lower are the costs and the better the health status of the population (Starfield and Shi 2002).

Simultaneously the WHO rightly identified poverty as the major underlying and fundamental public health threat. How poverty and related social injustice impacts on vulnerable groups soon becomes obvious in the public health sphere (Starfield 2001; Starfield and Shi 2002). The global number of people estimated to be infected or at risk of schistosomiasis has not been reduced over the last 50 years but 85 per cent of those affected are the poor in Africa (Engels *et al.* 2002). This may well explain the lack of effective international action. Childhood TB is a growing problem in some parts of the world and is out of control (Donald 2002). It is estimated that 1 million children each year are forced into prostitution worldwide and that at any one time there could be 10 million child prostitutes and yet this major public health problem does not receive proper attention (Willis and Levy 2002). Again the victims will usually come from the poorest parts of the world, the poorest groups in those societies or those marginalised in society. Mental ill-health is a major global problem but still much neglected (Davis 2002). Road traffic injuries are a global public health problem (Peden and Hyder 2002) but the victims lack the power of the global vehicle manufacturing industry who often dominate national government transport planning. The political and economic power base in the world has not altered and that is proving to be one of the major obstacles to effective global public health policy and practice (Legge 2002).

In the twenty-first century there have been challenges to some deep-rooted determinism and parochialism and at times narrow nationalism in some sectors of public health. There is an increasing recognition that simply because life expectancy is rising in the northern hemisphere, there is no certainty that it will always continue to do so. If it does, there will be enormous public health implications in terms of demands on health and social services, planning, pensions and so on. However, at a global level the old threats to public health are still very much present and take an enormous toll of the world's population with women and children bearing the greatest human costs. Linked to major public health problems of food, water and shelter, evidence has emerged about the aggressive marketing of tobacco by northern countries not only in Africa and Asia but also Central and Eastern Europe. Globally at least 15 per cent of all cancers are estimated to be due to smoking and 'this figure is expected to increase because of the uptake of tobacco use in low-income countries' (Kuper *et al.* 2002).

The critical importance of poverty as a determinant of health must be addressed by quite sophisticated and complex programmes that translate economic programmes to reduce and remove poverty into effective public health advances (Braveman *et al.* 2002). These programmes must also be linked to sustainability. They may be achieved in some respects far more rapidly in terms of their impact on global public health through food and water security programmes than for instance through North American or Northern European programmes. In these latter regions, economic interventions to improve public health by reducing poverty are mediated by overt and covert economic influences of the tobacco, food, alcohol, air polluting and climate warming industries. In the United States, consumers in 2002 are contemplating action against junk food manufacturers whose products they consider have wrecked their health and their lives in a country where 61 per cent of adults are estimated to be overweight and where the economic costs of obesity will be $117 billion in 2000 (Charatan 2002; PA News 2002). So the United States estimates that 400 000 of its citizens die each year from tobacco-related diseases and around 300 000 will die from obesity and weight-related diseases. Globally cardio-vascular diseases are escalating (Reddy 2002).

Public health has been undertaken for the public and on the public. One of the major new challenge for practitioners may be to explore more fully than has hitherto been the case, the possibilities of doing public health with 'the public' (Wang 1975; Rosenthal 1982; Stark 1985; Soori and Motlagh 1999; Ramos *et al.* 2001; Swider 2002; Umar 2002). Public health worker as advocate has long been mooted, public health worker as facilitator and supporter of public interventions in public health is perhaps the ultimate challenge and may require the development of or focus on existing or new skills. This challenge for practitioners is linked to working out effective strategies that will ensure actions on addressing inequalities in public health become meaningful. User and community groups have untapped knowledge and understanding of many public health issues relating to exposures, effects, access to services, social support, impacts of social exclusion, good practice and so on. The societal challenge will be to tap into and use that knowledge and understanding far more than has hitherto been the case and the professional challenge will be to ensure that even more public health staff recognise the value of such a process and do not feel threatened by it.

The contributors to this book have shown primarily but not exclusively in the UK context how public health practice can effectively benefit local and regional, rural and urban, community and workplace health. They describe the technical, organisational and managerial skills needed to impact upon health. Progress may be limited or can be substantial but it is possible in every field covered by the book. It is most effective when it fully engages the public (Barker *et al.* 2002). The problems and challenges that remain are, however, enormous. Without substantial political commitment and action the practitioners and public will not be able to ensure the national and global progress in public health that is still urgently needed.

References

Barker RD, Millard FJ and Nthangeni ME (2002) Unpaid community volunteers – effective providers of directly observed therapy (DOT) in rural South Africa. *S Afr Med J* **92**(4): 291–4.

Braveman P, Starfield B and Geiger HJ (2002) World Health Report 2000: how it removes equity from the agenda for public health monitoring and policy. *BMJ* **323**: 678–81.

Butler C (2002) Globalisation and Health. Those concerned with health must continue to challenge power. *BMJ* **324**: 1276.

Charatan F (2002) Lawyers poised to sue US junk food manufacturers. *BMJ* **324**: 1414.

Davis NJ (2002) The promotion of mental health and the prevention of mental and behavioural disorders: surely the time is right. *Int J Emerg Ment Health* **4**(1): 3–29.

Donald PR (2002) Childhood tuberculosis: out of control? *Curr Opin Pulm Med* **8**(3): 178–82.

Engels D, Chitsulo L, Montressor A and Savioli L (2002) The global epidemiological situation of schistosomiasis and new approaches to control and research. *Acta Trop* **82**(2): 139–46.

Feacham RGA (2001) Globalisation is good for your health, mostly. *BMJ* **323**: 504–6.

Feacham RGA (2002) Globalisation is good for your health, mostly. *BMJ* **324**: 44.

Horton R (2001) Ghana: defining the African Challenge. *Lancet* **358**: 2141–9.

Kuper H, Adami HO and Boffetta P (2002) Tobacco use, cancer causation and public health impact. *J Inter Med* **251**(6): 455–66.

Legge D (2002) Challenge of globalisation deserve better than simplistic polemics. *BMJ* **324**: 44.

PA News Friday 14 June 2002. Fast Food Giants fund anti-obesity campaign.

Peden M and Hyder A (2002) Road traffic injuries are a global public health problem. *BMJ* **324**(7346): 1153.

Ramos IN, May M and Ramos KS (2001) Environmental health training of promotoras in colonias along the Texas–Mexico border. *Am JPH* **91**(4): 568–70.

Reddy KS (2002) Cardiovascular diseases in the developing countries: dimensions, determinants, dynamics and directions for public health action. *Public Health Nutr* **5**(1): 231–7.

Rosenthal MM and Greiner JR (1982) The barefoot doctors of China: from political creation to professionalization. *Hum Organ* **41**(4): 330–41.

Soori H, Motlagh E (1999) Iranian rural health workers (behvarz) and risk factors of childhood injury. *East Mediterr Health J* **5**(4): 684–9.

Starfield B (2001) Improving equity in health: a research agendas. *Int J Health Serv* **31**(3): 545–66.

Starfield B and Shi L (2002) Policy relevant determinants of health: an international perspective. *Health Policy* **60**(3): 201–18.

Stark R (1985) Lay workers in primary health care: victims in the process of social transformation. *Soc Sci Med* **20**(3): 269–75.

Swider SM (2002) Outcome effectiveness of community health workers: an integrative literature review. *Public Health Nurs* **19**(1): 11–20.

Umar US, Olumide EA and Bawa SB (2002) Voluntary health workers' knowledge, attitude and practices regarding record keeping in Akinyele LGA of Oyo State, Nigeria. *Niger Postgrad Med J* **9**(1): 17–22.

Wang VL (1975) Training of the barefoot doctor in the people's Republic of China: from prevention to curative services. *Int J Health Serv* **5**(3): 475–88.

Weisbrot M, Baker D, Kraev E and Chen J (2002) The scorecard on globalization 1980–2000: its consequences for economic and social wellbeing. *Int J Health Serv* **32**(2): 229–53.

Willis BM and Levy BS (2002) Child prostitution: global health burden, research needs and interventions. *Lancet* **359**(9315): 1417–22.

Index